"Ask me what this book is about and I will struggle to give you a simple answer. It is about pregnancy and birth, anxiety and despair, blood and water. It is memoir and history, poetry and theology. Ask me, though, why you should read this book, and my answer is very simple—because you are a person with a body in and through which you bear pain, fear, and failure. Read this book for its necessary wisdom. In our most desperate vulnerability, when all we can do is endure, God is there too."

Ellen Painter Dollar, author of *No Easy Choice: A Story of Disability, Parenthood, and Faith in an Age of Advanced Reproduction*

"*Birthing Hope* drew me in from the first page to the last. Rachel Marie Stone's masterful interweaving of family story, theological truth, and personal reflection on birth, life, and loss puts her in the company of writers such as Rebecca Solnit and Eula Biss. I will return to this book for wisdom, beautiful writing, and encouragement that, even in the face of loss and sorrow, it is good to give ourselves to the light."

Amy Julia Becker, author of *Small Talk* and *A Good and Perfect Gift*

"We all carry fear with us in our bodies. Some of us try to escape it, some excel at denying it, and others attempt to bully it into submission. Rachel Marie Stone's shimmering writing instead invites readers to recognize the ways in which fear shapes us (and sometimes breaks us) as human beings. *Birthing Hope* reveals, with honesty and grace, the ways in which holy, embodied hope can re-form our response to fear."

Michelle Van Loon, author of *Moments & Days: How Our Holy Celebrations Shape Our Faith*

"Rachel Stone writes with power in this captivating reflection on the legacies of pain, procreation, and promise that echo through women's (reproductive, emotional, and familial) lives. Part memoir, part travelogue, part time travel, *Birthing Hope* kept me glued to its pages. Highly recommend!"

Jennifer Grant, author of *Love You More*, *Wholehearted Living*, and *Maybe God Is Like That Too*

"I've been waiting for a book like this one for years, and no one could have written it more beautifully and wisely that Rachel Marie Stone. With the skill of a poet and the patience of a doula, Stone invites the reader to look straight into the face of fear and find in it the spark of hope. There are words and phrases from these pages that I will go on pondering for years. Theologically rich and carefully researched, *Birthing Hope* is a book for everyone, but as a new mother it proved life changing—the kind of book that leaves you breathless."

Rachel Held Evans, author of *Sec⸻ ⸻ ⸻ Biblical Womanhood*

"Every woman who gives birth knows that it is a profoundly spiritual experience. Something in us changes as our bodies bring life into the world. Rachel Marie Stone puts words around the ways the birthing process pulls women into the depths of pain, but also identity, fear, mercy, and even death. In doing so, she offers a clear look at the physical, emotional, and mystical messiness of birth."

Carla Barnhill, author of *The Myth of the Perfect Mother*, former editor of *Christian Parenting Today*

"Profound theology, deep psychic insight, and the kind of wisdom that only emerges from immersion in life and the Scriptures—Rachel Marie Stone's book is a treasure, unforgettable, entirely compelling."

James Howell, author of *Worshipful: Living Sunday Morning All Week*

"Why do so many movies and TV shows portray birth so laughably poorly? It's as if we've all agreed the real thing—the most elemental human reality—is too raw and inelegant, too terrible and ecstatic, to be honest about. Rachel Marie Stone upends this conspiracy in this feisty, smart, theologically illuminating book. In her hands, birth is not only a sacrament of solidarity, a sign of hope amid the chaos of doubt and fright, but also a reminder that, for all our talk of immortal souls, we have and are bodies, fearfully and wonderfully so."

Wesley Hill, author of *Spiritual Friendship: Finding Love in the Church as a Celibate Gay Christian*

"*Birthing Hope* will plumb your depths and, if you let it, bring rise to something new in you. Reading this book, I rediscovered pieces of me I had hidden away, dusted them off, and found that they were now different from when I had last concealed them. These are powerful words crafted by a tender heart and hands. Rachel Marie Stone has written a book for our souls. I urge you to spend time with this book."

Michael Wear, author *of Reclaiming Hope: Lessons Learned in the Obama White House About the Future of Faith in America*

"I love this book. You needn't have given birth to love it. Maybe you don't even have to be curious about God or life as a human being to love it—the prose is that strong and compelling that perhaps even the God-and-human-uncurious might love it. My copy is going on my read-once-a-year shelf, after Jane Smiley and before Robert Penn Warren."

Lauren F. Winner, associate professor at Duke Divinity School, author of *Wearing God*

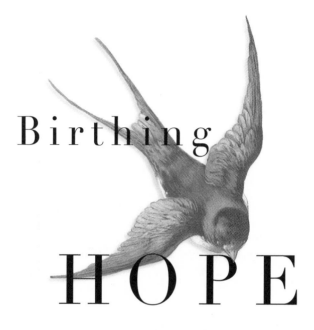

Birthing

HOPE

GIVING FEAR TO THE LIGHT

Rachel Marie Stone

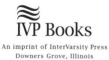

IVP Books

An imprint of InterVarsity Press
Downers Grove, Illinois

InterVarsity Press
P.O. Box 1400, Downers Grove, IL 60515-1426
ivpress.com
email@ivpress.com

InterVarsity Press® is the book-publishing division of InterVarsity Christian Fellowship/USA®, a
movement of students and faculty active on campus at hundreds of universities, colleges, and schools of
nursing in the United States of America, and a member movement of the International Fellowship of
Evangelical Students. For information about local and regional activities, visit intervarsity.org.

Scripture quotations, unless otherwise noted, are from the New Revised Standard Version of the Bible,
copyright 1989 by the Division of Christian Education of the National Council of the Churches of Christ
in the USA. Used by permission. All rights reserved.

While any stories in this book are true, some names and identifying information may have been changed
to protect the privacy of individuals.

"Rachel Cried There for Her Children" by Rivka Miriam is from These Mountains: Selected Poems of
Rivka Miriam (Jerusalem: The Toby Press, 2009). Used by permission.

"Darkness" by Micha Boyett is used by permission of the author.

Cover design: Cindy Kiple
Interior design: Jeanna Wiggins

Images: flying bird: Swedish greetings card, Swedish School / Private Collection / © Look and Learn /
Valerie Jackson Harris Collection / Bridgeman Images
bird's nest: © Onimages/iStockphoto/Getty Images

ISBN 978-0-8308-4533-0 (print)
ISBN 978-0-8308-8701-9 (digital)

Printed in the United States of America ∞

InterVarsity Press is committed to ecological stewardship and to the conservation of natural resources in
all our operations. This book was printed using sustainably sourced paper.

Library of Congress Cataloging-in-Publication Data
A catalog record for this book is available from the Library of Congress.

P	19	18	17	16	15	14	13	12	11	10	9	8	7	6	5	4	3	2	1
Y	34	33	32	31	30	29	28	27	26	25	24	23	22	21	20	19	18

FOR MY FOREMOTHERS:

Kitty and Lena and Goldie and Jennie;

Charlotte and Peggy.

AND FOR MY MOTHER:

Jeanette.

CONTENTS

DARKNESS

We are all some mother's child,
all born through great pain,

then a flood of release, an unbearable empty.
I sang a broken song, a wail of psalm

until you came. We were cold, alone,
this man who will raise you, and I.

No mother, no midwife, one blanket
a borrowed pot of water on the fire.

Did I not expect you would cry with me,
you who had willed every infant's cry?

Did I not expect you would need me,
your body suddenly cold, craving my skin?

You bobbed your head along my chest
in search of milk: ordinary, human.

Where were the trumpets, where the showering
of gold? We three were hushed in the dark,

my blood trickling to the ground, my husband's silent tears,
your infant body learning to swallow.

And in this, somehow, Glory.

My God, you deserve more than the two of us,
torn open and shivering with you in the dark.

MICHA BOYETT

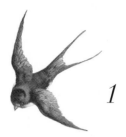

1

FLOAT

Spanish-English

DAR A LUZ
transitive verb phrase (idiomatic)

To give birth. (Literally "to give to light.")

In the beginning, there were the waters, and the Spirit of God moved lightly over the surface of the waters, and the dark, deep waters rippled and trembled with the movement of God.

And God gave all that is to light. And God called all of these things good: the light, and all that the light shone on, and all that is in the depths of the waters that the light did not shine on.

Tov. Good, God said.

I trembled and clung to my father's neck by the apartment pool and would not consent to be taken into the water. He said he would hold me the whole time, but going into the water, even in his arms, was unthinkable. I was sure we could not pass through it and live to tell. The photographs of my baptism, in the Sea of Galilee, when I was seven, show me smiling, but with spindly arms and legs all right-angled, tensed and clinging to my father's arms as he immersed me— *you are buried with Christ in baptism*—and raised me, spluttering seawater; eyes squeezed tight against the brilliant Middle Eastern sun. I could not yet swim.

Until I was eight, I lived in New York City. Now and then my parents and I went and stayed for a few days at the small beach cottage way out on Long Island, built by my dad's grandma, my grandma's mother, the year that my dad was born. It sat among the native vegetation, all scrubby pines and dune grasses, full of pale buttery light, and the sounds of the Atlantic's waves through the open windows: no frills but these. The surf was rough, too rough, by my parents' estimation, for swimming. I dug holes, sculpted sand, hunted beach glass, and let the waves bury my toes with sand at the high edges of the tide. When the waves were rough, I ran in terror, as had my father before me, in his childhood summers spent on that beach.

One summer, my mother brought her sewing machine to the beach house and made a dress at the same sturdy table that had held dozens of summertime meals, clusters of sun-pinked children gnawing corn on the cob and mincing their overcooked hamburgers—which they called "meat cakes"—into bits, which they mixed with ketchup as lubrication. An only child, I sat in the white wicker rocker with the huge spring cushion, reading book after book, and waiting to go down to the sea again, and begging to go see the dead whale.

The whale had washed up dead on the shore and stank with a terrific stink. It was also unimaginably large, especially by my lights. I couldn't stop myself from looking at it, from taking in the awful stench of it, the massive size of it. A living thing so enormous was a part of this world, just as I was, and other living things, huger and stranger, occupied the dark vastness of the ocean, which, from there on the beach, was beyond endless for all I could see. Now the whale was dead, stopped, just lying there and rotting and fertilizing my imagination. *What kind of whale was it? What did it die of? What will they do with it now?* I asked questions until my parents, worn by my incessant inquiry and not in possession of any further knowledge of this whale or whales in general, said I wasn't allowed to talk about it any more. Had there been a children's adaptation of *Moby-Dick* on the beach house's plentiful shelves, I might have buried myself in it, but instead my

3

mind itched, reaching for information and for a narrative when there was only a presence (the whale) and an absence (its life) wrapped in mystery and malodorous blubber. I could think of little else.

We moved from New York City to Eastern Long Island, in a house facing not the wild Atlantic, but the largely becalmed Peconic Bay. A short walk in almost any direction led to beaches or docks: on one side, the bay, on the other, the Long Island Sound. Still I feared water. These waves slapped lazily at rocky beaches, cresting and breaking only on exceptionally windy days. I collected rocks resembling food—lamb chops, baked potatoes, peas—or else tried to skip flat, smooth rocks across the surface, once, twice, thrice, the way my dad did so effortlessly. I dug many deep holes, and mostly avoided getting wet.

Once, I was playing with a small group of children at a calm swimming spot on the bay. Schools of minnows swirled in the shallows, so thick they could be scooped up in a plastic pail. I gathered a pail of them and nestled the pail's bottom in the sand, in a spot in the sun so I could see the minnows well—fragile-looking fish lips like the buttonholes of a filmy silk blouse, gaping and pursing, little rainbows playing off their scales; tiny black eyes somehow serious.

I could look at minnows for hours, just as I could play with one patient ladybug for the better part of a summer's day, letting it hike over the tall grass of my arm hair, tickling its way to my shoulder, from which I'd transfer it to the other hand and so on. One afternoon, I cried when my dad asked me to leave my ladybug in the garden outside the nursing home, where we had come to visit the elderly. He was the Baptist pastor in the small town, and some of the old saints now resided at San Simeon, by the Long Island Sound. He relented.

Just keep the bug. Try not to let anyone see that you've got it.

I wandered the halls, shaking hands and smiling and receiving kisses and listening to half-remembered stories, all in the secret, pleasant company of my ladybug. We always washed our hands before we left: my dad explained, well out of earshot, that when people got very old, they might not remember to wash their hands after they went to the bathroom. So we washed ours. My ladybug rode home in the car in my hand. Later, in the yard between home and church, it flew away, and I felt a twinge of loneliness and loss. I said goodbye, as I always did. It wasn't kind to hold on to wild things, I knew.

I would have liked to take the minnows home that day, but they'd have died in short order had I tried that. As I studied my minnows, some of the other children began digging holes and pouring buckets of minnows into them, covering them quickly with sand. They laughed. I screamed at them, tears hot in my eyes.

You're killing them for no reason! Stop it!

They stared, stunned by my fury, but perhaps also amused at my carrying-on and annoyed that I was taking their fun so seriously. A grownup left her beach chair to investigate, and told the other kids to stop.

I was aware of my own drama and enjoyed it a bit: casting myself in the role of heroic minnow savior. But I was also sick at heart, thinking of those little buttonhole mouths gasping their last in the rocky sand. Images like that stuck with me for days: an injured pigeon, a limping dog, a dead deer. A dark, cavernous hollow would open inside me, and I sensed doom. One evening, as I walked my dog around the yard, she barked and lunged at a stray cat, who made for the other side of the street and was hit and killed before my eyes. I couldn't look at my dog for days, and the moving picture of the scared cat flying dead from under the tires played on a repeating loop in my head.

"I'd rather just go to the Lewises' pool," I'd whine, when my parents brought up the question of my learning to swim. I didn't swim there, either—just bobbed around in an inflatable ring in the shallow end once arm floaties and goggles and nose clip had all been secured. These layers of protection were embarrassing, since all the other kids were playing Marco Polo and swimming in the deep end, apparently not fearing death by drowning. I fantasized about an ordinary bathing suit with floatation pads discreetly sewn inside it—it would hold me up, and it might make me look portly, but I'd look more like the other kids, and I wouldn't have to learn to swim.

My mom said I'd have an easier time learning to swim if I tried it at the beach. *Salt water helps with buoyancy*, she said.

I knew this; we'd visited the Dead Sea in Israel, and I watched as our friends waded in and then stretched out, heads lifted, as the sea lifted them high, like ducks. I dipped my feet in but went no further. "Dead" Sea is a creepy name, and the water was milky with salt, not quite transparent. Who knew what might be lurking beneath?

I like pools better, I told my mom. *With a pool, you can see to the bottom. You know nothing is under there about to get you.*

My dad was sympathetic. He didn't learn to swim until he was twenty-seven; when he was a child, his own father had dragged him, screaming, into the roaring Atlantic, which didn't exactly eliminate his fear of water. As he did with other things that terrified me—Ferris wheels, summer camp, roller-skating—my dad didn't push. But everything that scared me also attracted me. I pictured myself gliding along the lake on water skis, but couldn't get out of the boat; I imagined taking off across the skating rink gracefully, but always clung miserably to the rails along the perimeter. I was the crying, runny-nosed child for whom the carnival ride operator had to stop the roller coaster she thought she could brave.

Eventually, I doggy paddled, without even the arm floaties, along the shallow end of the pool. The next summer, I was swimming. Later, feet encased in protective neon-colored water shoes, I braved the calm waters of the Peconic Bay, where the occasional jellyfish or unseen pinching crustacean or imaginary sea monster would scare me ashore, sometimes for the remainder of the season. But I learned to scamper and swim quickly out of the shallows to where my feet no longer touched. I'd stretch out my arms and arch my belly to the sky, closing my eyes to the sun, enjoying the sea-muffled beach sounds of gulls and children and tubular aluminum-frame beach chairs screeching open. In those moments I felt I was being held in the womb of the earth. I exhaled forcefully, to see if I could make myself sink. Instead the waters, or the Lord, held me like a babe in arms, rocking, rocking; giving me again and again to the light.

Our first voyage is a watery one. Deep within a woman's body, in the darkness, cells divide again and again. Once, there was almost nothing; nothing that looked like much, but tended and guarded in that watery dark, the fragile, near-invisible almost nothing became you. Your mother's blood, and maybe her bones, fed you. Constantly you were held and rocked; you were never alone, never hungry, never dirty. Your mother was herself your food, your clothing, your shelter, your breath. She grew large, grew tired, grew uncomfortable. Then the water that held you trembled with a movement that came not just from her but through her, and, one way or the other, you came to light: wet with water and marked with your mother's blood.

Then you felt cold or hot or hungry or alone; perhaps you remembered, then, the time before, when you floated weightless, but you contended with gravity now; your limbs had a troubling freedom. You learned to fear and to be comforted, to get your hands dirty and then to wash them, to walk and then to fall, and to walk again.

Birth, and many of the things that precede and attend and are implied by birth, provides potent, formative, and enduring metaphors, which is perhaps another way of saying that many stories can be told as birth stories. Birth is a metaphor for creative work, for risks worth taking, for pain that resolves into joy, for new beginnings, for struggle that is rewarded. Our language links thought itself with that which precedes birth—conception. A person who helps an idea or a process along its journey (and birth is a journey) is sometimes likened to a midwife; when we mean to communicate how vulnerable we feel, we speak of assuming the fetal position. Also implied in birth, though these metaphors are less commonly discussed, are connection and separation, community and individuality, risk and sacrifice, life from death, darkness that gives way to light.

I have read that a woman's body acquires cells from each of the babies she carries, even as early as seven weeks into pregnancy. Those cells become part of her brain, part of her kidneys, even part of her beating heart. Scientists say that this may be protective, a boon to health; or it may be harmful, a contamination. This biological phenomenon seems merely to confirm what many women speak of as emotional and metaphorical experience: the sense that children, and even pregnancies that do not result in living children, change you, stay with you, become part of you in one way or another, in ways that are joyful and intimate, and in ways that are painful and intrusive.

So too do all our journeys and endeavors and relationships leave their marks, for better and worse. To bring anything new into the world is to open one's self and therefore to take on risk, to contaminate oneself with the other, to be made vulnerable. This requires not just courage but many things, among them faith, hope, help, companionship, grace—in a word, love. But if what we seek is fertility—if we seek productive power, fruitfulness, generativity—we cannot maintain sterility; we dare not, therefore, be too protective. Sex that's potentially generative of babies is sometimes referred to as unprotected. Unprotected is more or less what we need to be when we dare to create or to love. Bringing something new to light requires us to dive fully into the water.

This book is about that plunge.

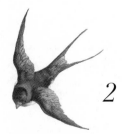

RISK

Spanish-English

LO SIENTO
(verb phrase)

I'm sorry. (Literally "I feel it.")

On the wall of the break room hung a hand-drawn, unfinished bar graph. The last entry, from a year or two prior, showed the number of women who had died that month, during or shortly after childbirth, in that hospital. There were perhaps sixteen or eighteen months represented, though I don't remember how many deaths it recorded, only that there were no months with no deaths. The graph was rendered in marker, and its maker had clearly taken great care in its preparation, using a meter stick to mark the lines and tidy penmanship to record the details. But it hadn't been finished.

There were other posters on the walls; some in Chichewa, the most commonly spoken language in that region of Malawi, and some in English, the language brought by the British. Some posters bore the symbol of USAID with the declaration "from the American people," which always swelled my throat with homesickness and pride. The posters advised various things in word and image. One declared that everyone, no matter how wealthy or poor, should ascertain their HIV status. Another reminded health care workers that antiretroviral drugs should always be given to pregnant women to prevent mother-to-child transmission. Still others explained that rape was an illegal crime, not a marital right.

Beads of sweat snaked their way down my back. My dark green scrubs, which had been custom-made by a tailor near the open-air market, were polyester, and, like most clothing of synthetic fiber, they turned my own perspiration against me. I itched, flushed with heat and with creeping anxiety. Circling the break room again, I took in the sagging, torn vinyl couches, the tattered carpet, the general dimness and grimness in contrast to the polished desk and pleasant lighting in the air conditioned office of the hospital's director, who, on the strength of a few recommendation letters on my behalf and a membership card from an American doula certification program, had agreed to let me observe the workings of the parts of the hospital serving women. I gazed at the hand-drawn chart again. Maybe the only thing sadder than a small hospital racking up maternal death each month is when that hospital gives up logging those deaths. The graph told no particular story beyond this: babies keep being born and women keep dying. Sometimes more, sometimes fewer, and never in a predictable pattern.

On the other end of my cell phone, my mother chatted about her plans for Easter weekend. I'd only been half-listening, consumed as I was with itchy sweat and the gloominess of the break room. Though I was old hand at spending holidays far from my family—my husband and I had lived two years in California, three years in Scotland, and a year in Germany before coming to Malawi—I never felt such longing for home as I did during holidays, and especially as I did just then. Last year, my mom and I planted eggs and bunnies and chicks around the same yard where I had played on a swing set and collected ladybugs and buried beloved pets. Later, the boys ran through the garden in their pajamas, sneakers pulled on hurriedly, announcing the Easter bunny's bounty so loudly that we shushed them not to wake the neighbors.

I couldn't recreate that in our Malawian garden, where any suggestion of sweetness anywhere instantly rallied armies of bugs and other crawly things, which were adept even at squiggling their way into apparently sealed packages. Leave a factory sealed bag of oats in the pantry long enough and you might later find fully grown moths rattling the bag in a quest for freedom. The Easter bunny would come, but he'd leave the goodies in a Ziploc bag on the dining room table, shortly before dawn.

As my mom talked about the Good Friday service, and what she'd bought for Easter dinner, I rolled my neck this way and that, trying to stop the tears rising in my eyes. I lifted my hands to the dull overhead light and examined my almost-healed paper cut, my many hangnails, my always torn and chewed cuticles. *Does this count as broken skin*, I wondered. I pulled a small bottle of hand sanitizer from my pocket and slathered my hands for the third or fourth time, accepting the alcohol's sting as (I hoped) purifying.

"Honey?" My mom finally noticed that I hadn't said much. "Are you okay?"

"I'm okay. I just miss you. And Greenport. And . . ." my voice wavered. "I want to go home."

"How many hours have you been at the hospital today?"

"No, I mean, I want to come *home*."

"I know, honey, I know you do." She spoke as if to a child.

I said I had to get back to the ward, and we promised to talk later, maybe, if the time difference allowed. We talked every day. Most days, I white-knuckled it to noon or 1 p.m., when it would be 5 or 6 a.m. for her and I could finally call. Maybe it would have been better if, like missionaries of old, I'd packed all my possessions in my coffin and set out to live and end my days there—scuttling the ships like Hernán Cortés and his conquistadors in the land of the Aztecs, who, for vastly different reasons, severed all ties to the Old World and obliterated the possibility of retreat. As a child I'd send letters and packages to a missionary nurse my church supported in West Africa; I thought I might grow up to be like her, happiest tending to the wounds of the poorest of the poor. Dear missionary Sarah couldn't wait for her furlough to end so she could return to her rustic dispensary. I had email and Facebook and a cell phone that kept the people and places I longed for on the other side of the globe virtually before my eyes and ears on a daily basis, and though I was glad for these, I suspected they also prevented me from being entirely *there*.

I slipped my phone into my pocket and headed back to the ward, which was at least brighter than the break room thanks to its large, open windows. Despite the prevalence of malaria, the windows were screenless. Dingy curtains, gray with grime, hung limply, not drawn. Husbands were not allowed to accompany their wives on the labor-and-delivery ward for reasons of "modesty," but male employees of the hospital—doctors and nurses and orderlies and janitors—

could be seen and heard a few feet away from the metal-framed beds where women lay struggling their babies into the world.

"Come over here," Kennedy, a young male student midwife, called to me. He wanted help. Despite my reminders that I was not a midwifery student and was there only to observe, the midwives had enlisted me as a helper. The category of "doula" doesn't really exist as a doula in Malawi. I'd trained as a doula some years before, and I was here to see how childbirth and women's health were handed in this place—one of the poorest countries on earth and one of the worst in which to see birth. Already I'd seen a half-dozen or so babies born, and today I felt I'd seen enough. Now, as I stood with Kennedy and his patient, I fought revulsion and nausea as I watched the woman before me crying out in her pangs. Her body bore the evidence of female genital mutilation, perhaps also some venereal disease. The baby's head became visible. I wanted to run.

Normally, I loved being at births, though they are typically messy affairs. It gave me a high, like seeing a transcendent performance at the theater or a truly outstanding athletic feat: a woman struggles and shouts and endures, pushing her baby toward the light. The big bellies and the blood, the crying and the straining, and then, the sudden cleaving—the one body opening itself to the point of breaking to release this entirely separate being, emerging waxy-white and still, looking somehow ancient and new at the same time, eyes squeezed shut, arms rigid at the sides, then springing open, flailing, grasping, pinking themselves with a cry, squinting at the light and turning toward mama's voice as the mother herself reaches for the babe, glowing and transfigured, with triumph and love. Agony and ecstasy. It is the most bodily and most spiritual event I know. It is life touching hands briefly with death.

For several months, I'd been spending a few hours here and there in the various areas of the hospital dealing with women's health—the labor ward, but also the birth control clinic and the pre- and postnatal clinics, where, always, dozens of women waited and waiting, uncomplaining, for the brusque and often patronizing attentions of the uniformed nurses, who enjoyed their power and position. Some sneered at the women who were two days late for their quarterly contraceptive injections, ordering them to another all-day wait at the lab for a pregnancy test, or humiliating them by requiring them to show their menstrual blood. One barefoot, dusty, teary woman after another hitched up her skirts and pulled down what underwear or sanitary garment she had—usually just a rag tied around the waist with another rag tied fore and aft, passing between the legs. I perched at the midwife's desk, as I'd been told to. She handed me a ledger and a pen and instructed me to elicit and record information for each woman: name, date of birth, village, number of children, number of children still alive, HIV status. Women cried when the nurse refused them their contraceptive injections, sending them off without even condoms. Others winced at the jab of the needle before leaving, smiling and relieved—another three months without a pregnancy.

No one was quite sure why I was there, including me. I had ideas about training doulas in Malawi—Malawian women supporting other Malawian women in labor—but I was wary of sweeping in with ideas and advice. Too many white people have come to Africa brimming with good intentions; too many end up causing more harm than they could have anticipated. Characters like the hateful preacher in *The Poisonwood Bible* are rarer than the real danger: wonderfully compassionate and culturally sensitive missionaries and NGO workers who hurt where they mean to help, building houses and schools without employing local workers, handing out free clothes and shoes and thereby hurting businesses that sell secondhand clothes and shoes, distributing life-saving medicine in ways that make those who need them feel embarrassed and therefore mistrustful of modern medicine.

So I decided I'd observe for a while, since I was, after all, not a doctor or nurse but an English teacher and a writer. I'd watch without doing anything in particular. Eventually, maybe, I hoped, midwives and mothers would tell me what they needed, and maybe I'd be able to help with whatever that was. My Malawian neighbor Dahlia had said that a nurse holding her hand when she was struggling with a difficult labor had helped a lot, but typically, there was little hand-holding on the ward: not much time for it, and such "soft" practices didn't seem to be valued. So I tried to hold women's hands if I could, and, mostly, to stay out of the way. It was disquieting to discover that my white skin gave me *carte blanche*—deference I didn't deserve; all-access tickets into places I didn't have any business being.

But if Coca-Cola is here, I thought again and again, *then I want to be, too*. I felt sure that people like me, people from wealthy countries, needed to be here, needed to see. It seemed a good and sacred thing just to take in—to witness— all that that there was: beggars in the dirt, twisted legs folded underneath them, muscles wasted with disuse or eaten up by polio, women and girls sitting on grass mats for hours, plaiting one another's hair, the dance and laughter of ordinary conversation, the landscapes all brown and green and laced through with tall, elegant women, walking barefoot, robed in bright colors. I accepted the stares and the awkwardness of being the only white person in the church, in the room, in the market. I *should* feel like an outsider. In a graduate school class on postcolonial studies I learned about the paternalism that my mission training, later, would warn against. Watch and learn, suspend judgment and the impulse to intervene; meet people as people, as subjects of their own sovereign lives, not as objects and bit players in the drama of mine. I wanted to bear witness to what was here—this place so different from my home that it was hard to believe I'd taken an ordinary plane and not a space shuttle from New York City to land here; here, among people as much citizens of this earth as I.

Before the woman whose body repulsed me, before talking tearfully to my mother in the break room, I'd seen three babies born. The first was born to a very young woman so tired and week that she could barely lift her head to sip at the cloyingly sweet orange drink held to her lips. A crowd of young German medical students, here for a six-week international rotation, clustered around her bed and peered at her, earnestly. The midwife pushed synthetic oxytocin into an IV drip to speed the delivery. A fragile baby girl came, and the mother fell back on the bed, nearly expressionless.

The second baby was a hefty boy who came out of a woman who seemed neither young nor old. He burst forth from her with such a forceful gush of water and blood that the midwives leapt back, faces contorted with disgust and fear. The woman, who already had many children, smiled now that her baby was out and her ordeal over, and asked me to get her bag from under the bed, and to get out one of the new *chitenges* to wrap the baby in.

A *chitenge* is a two-yard cut of fabric, which serves, in much of sub-Saharan Africa, as skirt, shawl, baby carrier, blanket, and headwrap. New, they shimmered and glittered with colors of every rainbow hue. As they aged and wore out and became colorless and threadbare, they were ripped into makeshift underwear, diapers, and sanitary napkins, becoming, finally, something to be burned so that street dogs wouldn't coming nosing around for it. Just one *chitenge* easily cost a day's wages for someone who had a job aside from farming, so it must have been a sacrifice for this woman to buy several new ones to swaddle her baby, who, like most babies, would spend most of his first two years tied to her back in it.

In the preemie room, mothers used *chitenges* to bundle their too-tiny babies between their breasts ("better than incubator!" Lena, the head midwife, told me), and you'd often see newly-delivered women leaving the hospital, on foot, with day-old babies bundled and slung on their backs in *chitenges* ready for a five or six or ten mile walk to the village. Everywhere in Malawi you see this: babies tied on women's backs while they hoe fields and grind corn; babies tied on girl's backs, too, girls who are five or six years old, barely out of babyhood themselves. When I gave birth to my son in

California in 2005, "babywearing" was becoming a hip indicator of a certain kind of middle and upper-middle class parenting style; there were studies showing the benefits of the practice. Here it was just what it was.

Chitenges also served as sheets in the labor ward. All the mattresses in the ward were of brown vinyl and were sometimes draped with a sheet that appeared to have been rubberized once. Women in hard labor would spread one of their own *chitenges* over the bed to lie down on, but it would shift as they writhed in their pangs; invariably, their bare skin touched the vinyl and rubber, which could only have felt sticky and moist. I never saw anyone clean the mattresses. But the third laboring woman I saw that day lay down directly on it, with no *chitenge*, still fully clothed and clearly suffering.

"She has a long time to go yet." Chisomo, the midwife in charge that shift, was heavily pregnant herself. She sauntered back to the nurses' station to sip cold orange Fanta from a battered glass bottle and browse the newspaper. I tried to follow her, but the fully clothed woman reached and pleaded. I stayed. She grunted and moaned and called for her mother— *amayi! Amayi! Amayi!* Her *amayi*, with the other grandmothers, waited in a little dark alcove just outside; inscrutable rules prevented them being with their daughters. I spoke soothingly to her, looked into her eyes and tried to reassure her, but she was deep enough inside the lonely tunnel of late labor that words no longer had meaning. I think I held her hand, or she held mine.

"Help—over here!" I called to the midwives. The woman was hunching her shoulders, lifting her knees, and pushing.

"Come over, please!" I said, loudly, I thought, but as in one of those dreams where you try to scream but no sound emerges, no one seemed to hear.

The woman reached for the hem of her long black skirt. I helped her, throwing it back over her knees. There, facedown in a gathering pool of blood and water, was a baby. The woman didn't move to pick it up; she didn't seem to know it was there. My hands were bare, ungloved, and voices in my head argued with one another to the effect that I should do nothing, not being a midwife, but a louder voice from somewhere else told me to pick up that baby right away. I plucked it from the puddle beneath its mother's skirt, saw that she was a girl and that she was breathing, and lay her on her mother's chest.

"Here we use *gloves!*" The old midwife, Mayeso, shouted at me. I turned to the large slop sink and began scrubbing my hands with cold water—the only kind on tap—and the harsh green bar soap, again, all there was. There were no towels, paper or otherwise. Behind me, a woman pushed a pink-stained rag mop toward a drain in the floor. Mayeso watched me wash my hands, then demanded to see them.

"Do you have any cuts?"

My cuticles were always red and ragged and torn from my own nervous picking, and today they were as they always were. And I had a deep paper cut, but it had almost healed.

"Well, maybe," I said, looking at my battered fingers.

"Go show her!" Mayeso ordered, pointing me to Chisomo, who still sat at the nurses' station, paper in hand. She looked at my hands, bored.

"I'm sorry, I didn't mean to do it without gloves."

"Don't. Do it. Again."

Mayeso beckoned me to a small sink and poured a pint of disinfectant over my hands. I retrieved my hand sanitizer and slathered. Then Kennedy, who seemed to be doing most of the actual work that day, called me back to the woman whose baby I'd just grabbed. The woman smiled and laughed and gave me a high five, euphoric with her achievement.

"Can you help me open the sterile things?" Kennedy was getting ready to suture the woman's perineum, which had torn during the delivery. I snapped on gloves and carefully opened the sealed packets containing the suturing supplies in the order that Kennedy asked for them. By this day, perhaps only my fourth or fifth time at the hospital, I was no longer surprised that there would be no numbing medication to deaden the sensation of her flesh being sewn back together. The woman bit her lip and hugged her baby to her chest as the needle bit into her skin and Kennedy's still-learning hands fumbled a little with the sutures. With a free hand, I reached for hers and let her squeeze it as she swallowed the urge to cry out in pain. Chisomo, holding her own vast belly, came over to check Kennedy's work.

"These people on ARVs have such delicate tissue. Doesn't take much to tear and bleed," she observed, walking away again.

I felt my throat get tight and my shoulders draw up. Sweat tickled its way down from my armpits to my waist. Kennedy was finishing up.

"What's her *status*, Kennedy?" I asked.

"Reactive," he said, still looking down at his work. "She's HIV positive."

I pretended nonchalance. The woman's mother emerged from the dark little alcove and rushed to see her daughter and her daughter's first daughter, three generations of Malawian women. *To be born a woman in this country*, I thought. *Hard not to see it as a pity*. I mentally ran through dismal statistics on education and literacy and child marriage and sexual assault and maternal mortality and life expectancy for girls in this place. And yet these women rejoiced. *Here was life. Here was hope. It goes on.* I removed my gloves and washed my hands and the grandmother caught my hand and smiled.

But my smile was forced and my heart was cold. I was thinking of my nonintact skin and the virus, or viruses, that I'd touched. The baby would've been fine, probably, if I'd waited for one of the midwives to come over. What had I been thinking? I excused myself as quickly as I could and stood in the break room, staring at the posters full of statistics that I'd thought had nothing to do with me, and wondering how I managed to get blood on my hands when I was only supposed to be watching.

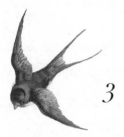

REFLECT

BLOOD

The red liquid that circulates in the arteries and veins of

humans and other vertebrate animals, carrying oxygen

to and carbon dioxide from the tissues of the body.

Family background; descent, lineage

IN ONE'S BLOOD
[phrase]

Ingrained or fundamental to one's character

I lay in my bed, crammed in with too many stuffed animals, and probed my itching chest with my fingers. Familiar dread started like heat and heaviness in my belly and cooled to a chill as it slithered up my back and gripped my throat. *Lumps. I feel lumps.*

Cancer. *Dear God, please don't let me die.* I began directing my funeral on the inner screen of my mind: my mother would wail loudly and fling herself into people's arms, and my father would save his tears for later, standing mostly silently, nodding and mouthing thanks to those who had come to mourn me. They would hand out little cards printed with my date of birth and date of death—just twelve years old!—and a picture of me smiling sweetly or gazing meaningfully into the middle distance, with a few lines of doggerel about how my death actually worked out to some sort of compliment—I was that special to God that I had to be transported to heaven on the express line.

I imagined the lovely flowers and my own corpse in its casket, and, before that, my deathbed scene, which had the elegance of a Victorian painting. There I would be in a beautiful white nightgown, in a bed made up all in white, tightly tucked, arms out and arranged prettily atop the blankets. I'd whisper goodbye, look toward the heavenly light beaming down on my pillow as a blue-eyed Jesus with wavy long hair smiled at me with very white teeth and extended his hand, and I'd close my eyes and fade away. It was pleasant to think of the nice things people might say about me once I was gone, but then I would remember that I would no longer *be*, and the hot-and-cold fear would creep back. My chest hurt and pricked. For days, every move and thought was edged with dread. If I forgot for awhile—immersed in a book or daydream—I would remember with a jolt, sobering up, morose, preparing to face my inevitable early demise.

Finally I told my mother. *Breast cancer, mom. I think have breast cancer.*

No, honey, that's just you becoming a woman. That's your bosom growing.

Don't tell daddy.

Then I went off and forced myself to play with my dolls, trying to stay a little girl; to arrest whatever it was that was coming to overtake me.

Another time, another part of my body was aflame with a mighty itch. I snuck a plastic baggie full of ice from the kitchen and brought it into the bathroom to cool the fire. I thought, sadly, about how whatever this was probably meant I'd never have children. I could see the doctor shaking his head. *You'll never become a mother*, he would say. *I'm so sorry.* I couldn't easily put this worry aside, since it lodged a constant reminder that finally grew so intense that I whispered a teary confession to my mother.

It's burning, you know, down there, I said, since there was and is no cute word I could use to talk about that part of my body, and to tell the truth, I was not entirely sure of what all

I actually did have below the belt. *Oh honey,* she said, *that's from the antibiotics you were on. It killed the good bacteria and let the bad take over. We'll get some yogurt.* Coffee-flavored Dannon and an over-the-counter cream soon quelled my physical discomfort and balanced the bodily flora, but my mind had already sculpted numerous expressways for dread and fear, and my mental traffic couldn't help but divert to their wide lanes, racing straight to the worst conclusions.

My mother grew up Jewish, nonobservant except for the ritual of bagels, nova salmon, and cream cheese on Sundays, and Chinese food on Christmas, with a little Hebrew school now and then, but she was in love with religion, and especially with Christianity, from the age of five or so, when her Irish Catholic nanny brought her along to mass. She enthusiastically greeted every habited nun she came across— *hi, Sister!*—and became devoted to Jesus at the age of sixteen, when eager, young evangelicals found her in a New York City park, smoking and cursing, and handed her a Gospel of John, which she read and loved. My father was half Irish and half French Canadian, a self-avowed atheist from the age of seven who nevertheless made First Communion and Confirmation in the Catholic Church at the usual times, only to become an evangelical Christian when he was in the military. By the time I was old enough to be aware of anything, the two of them belonged to a branch of evangelicalism that had a particular and awkward fondness for Jews, as Jews apparently figured into this evangelical end-of-the-world scenario in some important way.

All I understood though, was that even though we—that is, Jews, which I understood myself still somehow to be—were supposed to be God's chosen people, that mostly meant that pretty much from the day we existed people wished we didn't. And according to the hysterical evangelical newsletters that sometimes arrived in the church mail, even the death and destruction of the Holocaust was a drop in the bucket compared to what horrors were still coming for Jews before the end times. By third grade, I knew more about the Holocaust than many adults, and I sat at my little desk in Mr. Pekunka's classroom and thought about where I would hide when the Nazis came looking for me. It had nothing to do with my religion—I knew that plenty of Jews sought and received baptism only to travel right up crematoria chimneys. My blood, which I couldn't change, marked me for death.

These worries clung to the edges of my thoughts in both waking and sleeping like a kind of blackmail. *You thought you could forget about us and be a happy, regular kid*, the spooks whispered, *but don't forget about us! Don't forget about cancer and ghettoes and gas chambers! Don't forget about the end of the*

world and AIDS! For all the relative stability, security, and hap-
piness of my childhood there was a dread-filled counter-
weight—the certain understanding that it could all be taken
away in an instant, that it was all a historical and geographical
accident, that I might be bereft of all that made my life what
it was. Every time my parents left the house without me, I
was certain they would die in a car crash and leave me or-
phaned; I keened like a Sicilian widow if they were more than
five minutes late. The final layer to all this anxiety was my
awareness of how excessive and absurd it all was. I admon-
ished myself: *You have no reason to worry so much, and nothing
to be so upset over.*

Well, you come by it honest, my mom says. Travel along the
branches of our family tree and you find madness and de-
pression and stints in rehabs and asylums. My precocious
sense of dread may have been an atavism, a throwback to the
centuries during which my Jewish foremothers had endured
persecution and fled from pogroms, and those during which
my Irish foremothers endured malnutrition and dreaded the
British; centuries in which they all feared and mourned the
perils of childbirth and the illness and loss of infants and
children and loved ones. I have read that recent studies in
genetics are mapping the ways in which our ancestors' experiences are written into their genes. And it may have been a
learned behavior, too, those supposedly bygone fears never

really receding, even in the face of antibiotics and democracy and a relatively safe food supply. My mom is bipolar, and though I am not, I joke that I'm "bipolar curious"—up and down, happy and sad, sunshine and shadow, unlike my steady-state husband.

A recurring nightmare when I was in kindergarten and first grade went like this: My mom and I would be standing on the front stoop of a brick house in Brooklyn, a house much like our own, and My mom would ring the doorbell. At the same moment it was answered, she would lose control of her body functions, sneezing and coughing and crying and more, all at once. I always awoke feeling ashamed. It was a dream about my mother losing control, and I couldn't let that happen. She'd been hospitalized when I was three, and I had mental snapshots: her lying in bed and sobbing for what seemed like days, her looking down at me in the lobby of the psychiatric hospital, my dad crying as he hugged me, the two of us alone in the apartment. That couldn't and wouldn't happen again. So I breathed shallowly, ground my teeth at night, clenched my shoulders during the day. Working off the principle that bad things happened to you when you least expected them to happen, especially *to you*, I developed, over the years, an elaborate ritual of worry, so that no bad thing could surprise me. This, the silent mental recitation of the Litany of Possible Horrors, was the approach to anxiety management favored by the Irish, maternal side of my father's family.

Before she left the house, my dad's mom, Grandma Peggy, would turn on the radio and shout "goodbye, Ralph," to her imaginary husband so as to fool the would-be burglars staking out the house. Her actual husband left her some years earlier with four children and precious little else, but she scraped together her intelligence, wit, and will, and went to work, sharing child-rearing with her mother, long retired, and her sister, on disability for mental illness. Grandma Peggy was tough. She gave birth so quickly and easily that she'd hammocked a towel between her legs on the way to the hospital because it felt like the babies were just going to tumble out, even my father, who weighed more than ten pounds and was born looking like a three month old.

Grandma Peggy always sniffed the milk before pouring it and taught me never to sleep in a hotel bed without underpants on under my nightie; someone she knew had gotten crabs doing that. She said "Ooh, Geez" a lot. Many things and people gave her the "fantods" or the "heebie-jeebies," and she had a nervous tic, a way of pursing and flexing her lips rhythmically. It looked to me like she was swishing mouthwash. She breathed heavily, snored loudly, and never bought store-brand or off-brand products; brand name only would do.

There were always flashlights, portable radios, extra batteries, and high-quality paper goods in her house.

Grandma Peggy carried with her everywhere an enormous handbag, which always held Snickers bars and Bounty paper towels (folded and placed in a Ziploc bag), an emergency whistle, and maybe a can of pepper spray. She said the chocolate bars were for Aunt Jane's low–blood sugar emergencies. Aunt Jane, the youngest of her children, was a juvenile diabetic, and grown and gone, but Grandma had gotten in the habit of carrying the candy, and it came in handy once when she pushed a piece of it into a stranger's mouth on the subway. Everyone thought that the man was drunk or crazy, but Grandma recognized the signs of insulin shock and saved the day.

Grandma Peggy's mother, Katherine, called Kitty, bought a piece of land on a sand dune, the only impulse purchase of her no-nonsense life, made one Sunday afternoon when she'd gone along with her sister on a drive out of the city. She built the house years later with the payout from the life insurance policy when her husband died, and thereafter gave her grandchildren grief about tracking sand into the house that she herself had built on a sand dune. Sometime in the mid-1970s, a rapist was said to have attacked in the vicinity, so Kitty made everyone sleep with the windows shut and locked, and supplied each individual with an air horn to be kept by the bed. Live on a sand dune but don't track in sand. Stay by the ocean but lock the windows, keeping out the rapists, yes, but also the cool, briny breeze and lulling roar of the Atlantic. Turn on the radio and shout goodbye to an imaginary man to fool the imaginary criminals. This thinking is as familiar to me as my own daydreams.

Grandma Peggy told me once that on her way to work she saw a man drop his drawers and deposit diarrhea on the sidewalk. *God, he probably had AIDS,* she said. *He was skinny and awful looking.* The time and place—New York in the late 1980s—made hers a pretty good guess. I wondered if I might end up as a bystander to a similarly disgusting episode and began extrapolating this fear to cover most public spaces. You never knew who might have bled or urinated on this very bit of sidewalk where you now stood. Urban legends about HIV-infected needles being positioned in movie theater seats or jabbed into unsuspecting strangers in crowds or strategically placed in the coin return slot of payphones were then in circulation, and it felt reasonable to assume that I was at risk, and to be on alert.

I was born the same year that a strange malady researchers called GRID first began killing gay men in New York and San Francisco. My mom received several pints of donated blood right after I was born, a few years before HIV was identified as the cause of GRID, which we now call AIDS, and before anyone realized that far from being restricted to the so-called "four Hs" generally regarded as contemptible "others" (heroin addicts, homosexuals, Haitians, and hemophiliacs), AIDS was indiscriminate. Statistically speaking, my mom wasn't in much danger, but she has sometimes mentioned those transfusions, aware that she wouldn't have been immune to the illness that so many religious people were then calling just punishment from God.

When I was five or six—not long after the first famous people started dying of AIDS and people finally started talking about the virus—my dad, who had been moderately unwell for several years, became acutely ill. He grew thin and gaunt. His mouth was lined with sores. He had diarrhea all the time. The members of our largely Italian church in Brooklyn, where he was the pastor, made lasagna and baked ziti. *Eat, eat*, they would say, *we have to fatten you up.*

But he got thinner and weaker. He lay on the couch in the middle of the day. He had generalized lymphadenopathy— swollen lymph nodes all over his body. He had unspeakable diarrhea. Once, I heard him crying in the bathroom. The doctors said it must be cancer, or it must be something else, but they didn't know what.

The Salvadoran grandmother of some church friends—known universally as *Mama*—spent two hours on the bus to come to our house, bearing a brown paper bag containing a single egg and several spices. *I make you* ponche de crema, *pastor. Ponche de crema make you better.* This was about all the English she could muster. It was basically warm eggnog, but the gesture was everything. An old woman giving what little she had to a sick man—her precious spices, her cherished ritual of care.

There was sickness in *Mama's* family, too—her granddaughter's husband was also sick, and no one could say with what. Joe was my dad's age, and the congregation offered prayers for them in the same breath. They were companions in illness, the "sick guys." Then one day, Joe, who was not gay, not Haitian, not hemophiliac, had an answer to what was wrong. He had once used needle drugs. Now his wife was infected.

My dad asked for the HIV test.

Joe and Vera lived by the water, and Joe had a glass bottom boat. He said he'd take me out on the bay, and that we'd be able to see the fish swimming underneath. Just a little while later, Joe was dead, and my dad's test came back negative.

It turned out to have been celiac disease—all that lovingly offered pasta full of the gluten that turned his body against itself. Bowls of rice replaced loaves of bread, and just a little while later, my dad was perfectly well, and the phone rang, and Vera, too, was dead.

My mother did not acquire the virus at my birth and did not pass it to me. My father did not have the virus and did not die, though he came close. We were okay, for now. But you never knew. Someone might rape you or poke you with a needle in a crowd or hide a needle in a movie theater seat. Someone might spill something disgusting on you. You might go for a dental cleaning only to be intentionally infected by a deranged hygienist.

Or, decades later, you might find yourself standing quite literally in the blood and body fluids of the maternity ward, holding your hands to the light and fretting over whether your chewed-up cuticles and paper-cut skin was broken enough to let in the virus you'd dodged all these years.

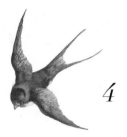

PREVENT

PREVENT
Verb (with object)

to keep something from happening

Origin

Late Middle English (in the sense "act in anticipation of"):
from Latin praevent—"preceded, hindered," from the verb
praevenire, from prae "before" + venire "come."

I was probably being dramatic, histrionic, even. Probably I just needed to go home, take a bath, have dinner and a beer, and forget about it. I meandered around the hospital's front entrance, taking in the long lines of people waiting for medicine, and the women waiting to have their babies weighed on a hanging scale in the open air, and the people bringing baskets of food for the patients. I'd be fine, I reasoned. My immune system was in good shape. The paper cut was really almost healed. My cuticles, well, they were battered, but it'd be okay. HIV dies after hitting the air anyway, doesn't it?

Then my husband, Tim, pulled up to the hospital gates in our rattling old Land Rover, our kids strapped in the seat behind him. I climbed in.

It was Good Friday, but I didn't have it in me to brave a service. We attended services at the Anglican church not only because we'd been gradually gravitating toward the Anglican tradition for years, when Tim was studying for his PhD in Scotland, but also because their services were predictable in length and comparably short. Moreover, the liturgy was already familiar to us from services in the United Kingdom and the United States. But the services at the Presbyterian church associated with the seminary where we taught could go on all day and followed unwritten liturgies we couldn't discern. Other expat families claimed that their children could sit quietly through hours of church, but Tim and I didn't want to do that to our kids or to ourselves. Some weeks, we didn't make it to services at all because one or more of us was ill, or in my case, either ill or suffering agoraphobia induced by culture shock, or both.

Sometime before I went to Malawi, I heard a missionary kid from somewhere in Africa tell a story about her mother:

the mother hadn't coped well with culture shock, and had instead spent many of her days locked in her bedroom, watching, rewinding, and rewatching a VHS tape of *The Sound of Music*. This story was meant to be funny, and I laughed, and because this was months before I found myself in the buzzing, confusing exhaustion of constantly navigating the unfamiliar, I imagined that I would never be so pathetic as to sequester myself with that cheerful, Europhilic confection of a musical. Then I found myself in Malawi, watching movies alone in bed, under the protective veil of mosquito netting, watching *The Sound of Music*, in fact, when even the thought of going outside made me tear up and sweat.

I've never had much of a poker face, so while I hadn't meant to say anything to Tim about the HIV positive woman and her baby and my gloveless, paper-cut, and raggedy-cuticle hands, he knew from the moment I climbed into the truck that something was up. I tried to play it cool, but my cheeks and ears were already glowing warm and pink.

"I mean, I didn't mean to do this, and I'm sure it's all going to be okay, but . . ."

"But what?"

"Well, this lady's baby kind of popped out right in front of me, and it was all face down in the birth water, and I thought it might drown or something before the nurse came over, so I grabbed it."

"Yeah, so what's wrong?" My husband has gutted elk. He's not so squeamish.

"Well . . . I didn't have gloves on. And I have a little paper cut, but it's really nothing because it's pretty much healed, but . . . turns out she's HIV positive . . . and I got her blood on my hands."

His knuckles whitened on the steering wheel and his voice grew higher.

"You're telling me that you have a cut on your hand, and you had no gloves on, and you picked up an HIV positive woman's baby and got her blood on your hands?"

"I'm sorry," I said, "I didn't mean to, since I didn't know she had HIV, and I thought the baby might die, even though it would've been fine. I wasn't being totally rational."

"You're right," he said, "That was not totally rational. I cannot believe this, Rachel! This is serious!"

"You're forgetting that HIV is so treatable. It's not a death sentence, you know."

"But that doesn't mean you go ahead and expose yourself to it!"

"Okay, I'll call Dr. Steinman when we get back and see what she says."

He was quiet then, staring at the road. As dusk gathered, visibility grew poor and he had to concentrate. It was hard to see the masses of pedestrians when it became dark. But he was also angry; I could tell. Or maybe he wasn't angry, but, like me, was afraid.

"I'm sorry," I said. "I'm so, so sorry."

He sighed and shook his head. "We need you to be okay," he said. "We need you."

I slipped off my shoes on the front porch and went straight for the washing machine, where I stripped to the skin and put everything I'd been wearing into the drum, pouring in a hefty measure of detergent. I washed my hands again and drew a scalding bath—we had no shower—scrubbing and scrubbing my arms, my scalp, my face, using a plastic bucket to pour water over my head, rinsing and rinsing again and again. I emptied the tub, filled it, and repeated the process. Then, still wrapped in a towel, I used our crummy mobile Internet device to log on to the website that let me call US numbers for next to nothing, and called Dr. Steinman, who'd given me her personal number when our son Graeme had been sick with malaria a few months prior. She was our travel medicine specialist in New York, and had given the four of us the many rounds of extra vaccinations a person needs in developing countries as well as prescriptions for antimalarial drugs and antibiotics we could self-administer in case of the inevitable onslaught of microbe-related gastric distress. An accomplished doctor and professor and a mother of four, she radiated intelligence and warmth, explaining the risks and rationales for each immunization and preventive medication. As she talked, I thought about how much safer it would be just to stay away from Malawi.

"I'm feeling stupid, Dr. Steinman," I said, when she came on the line. "I really just acted without thinking, and I got this woman's blood on my hands, and I have a paper cut that's pretty much healed, but . . ."

"Let me stop you one moment and see if I have this," she said. "So you picked up a baby that hadn't been washed or anything?"

"Right, it had just come out."

"And do we have any idea what drugs this woman might be on, if any, or what the viral load on her might be?"

"Not at all, I mean, I think she's on ARVs but I don't know which ones, or her counts."

Those kinds of diagnostics don't tend to exist for poor people in places like Malawi. If you have HIV, you get a combination of drugs. If it seems to work, you stay on that drug. If not, you try another one. You don't get to know your "counts."

"All right, here's what I recommend: you get yourself to the clinic ASAP and ask them for lamivudine and zidovudine—Combivir—and start taking it right away, unless they tell you that their PeP protocols call for a different combination. How many hours ago was this episode with the baby?"

"I think two? Too late to start PeP?" I knew that PeP—post-exposure prophylaxis—could prevent HIV infection, but that it had to be started soon after exposure, or it didn't work.

"No, it's fine. It's pretty good, actually."

"Ugh, I feel stupid. And worried."

Dr. Steinman sighed. "Let me tell you what," she said, sounding more like a friend than the earnest, cautious physician she was. "When I was in my residency—this is the late '80s—I was taking care of this guy with end-stage AIDS in the ICU. He was dying, but the family wanted us to pull out all the stops to keep him going. The viral load on this guy must have been tremendous. So the intern and I are trying to get a central line going, and he accidentally stabs me with the big needle. And we had none of the drugs. I couldn't relax until the tests came back clear, every six weeks for a year."

"Wow. Thank you for telling me that story."

"You're welcome. Get to the clinic."

It was growing dark in Zomba. I knew that Dr. Steinman, an observant Orthodox Jew, had only a few hours before the start of Shabbat. I thought of her lighting her candles, welcoming the Sabbath with a gentle stirring of the air, covering her eyes, rocking just a little, saying the prayers, breaking the challah and entering into sacred time. I felt calmed and grateful to know her, to have her on my side, on the other end of the phone, on the other side of the world.

I went to the clinic and asked for the drugs. The clinician asked a few questions, consulted a spiral-bound reference book, and handed me a large white bottle. I choked down the first of sixty large white pills as I stood in line to pay. I suppressed the urge to ask for extra pills, to take double doses, to drown my system in virus-inhibiting drugs.

At home I went online again, reading everything I could find about postexposure prophylaxis, the specific HIV drugs I was taking, and the effectiveness of the protocol. I read about the estimated risk of contracting the virus via blood splash over mucous membrane or "non-intact" skin. I looked up the medical definition of *non-intact* skin. Was my skin intact enough that the risk of exposure was actually zero? No, torn cuticles and almost-healed cuts were non-intact. I divided my statistical risk of infection by the estimated effectiveness of the PeP protocol to calculate the precise level of risk, which was something more than zero but something less than a tenth of a percent.

"I don't know how I'm going to live until I get the final results back in a couple of months," I said to Tim that night, as we lay under our mosquito net. "I thought I had to save the baby. It was almost instinctive, like my monkey brain said 'grab the baby' and I just did."

"Next time, try not to observe Good Friday so literally," he said, smiling his wry smile and putting his arms around me.

I didn't think I was a savior making a sacrifice, though. It just happened that I'd chosen to live in a place where a great many women of childbearing age were HIV positive, and in between trying to bear witness and to not be a bother, I'd barely touched the hem of suffering and illness that so many mothers here wore with a grace whose depths I could not fathom.

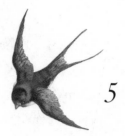

5

DIVE

Water idioms often highlight the dangerous or difficult
side of water. Here are 10 water idioms which
can help you describe difficult situations.

"To be in deep water: To be in a difficult
situation which is hard to deal with."

CHRIS MCCARTHY, "10 WATER IDIOMS
FOR DIFFICULT SITUATIONS"

I'd wanted to be a doula, in spite of the blood and sweat and poo in the birthing process, because I wanted to be near the miracle, and not just to read about it. I wanted to help other women ride the waves of childbirth. That's how I talk about getting through labor, but only if I'm asked. Assuming relative health and vigor—no small privilege—labor seems most endurable when you imagine each contraction coming in as a swell, washing over you, and receding; you find yourself falling into a rhythm that lets you ride each wave, one at a time. Some people talk about orgasmic birth or how birth can, with enough hypnosis or positive thinking or candlelight or yoga, be entirely painless, but they're usually selling something. As far as I can tell, nothing can take away the pain. You can't fight the ocean, or tame its billows, and trying will only exhaust you. All there is to do is ride the waves and keep your head mostly above the water. It's like being sucked into a rip current: you'll die of exhaustion if you fight it, but you'll live if you swim alongside it, letting it carry you until you and it part ways.

If it comes up that I gave birth to both of my children without medication, I'm quick to add that this wasn't actually a choice; forgoing the epidural was a choice made for me five years before my first child was born. A spinal operation had left my epidural space—the *dura mater* around my spinal cord—filled with scar tissue. My natural spine was twisted and twisting with scoliosis; in surgery, this was corrected and secured with a rod. This kept me from romanticizing the "natural" and from being able to receive an epidural. Without that option, my choices were these:

either be completely asleep—a C-section under general anesthesia—or be completely awake and feel everything. The intermediate option of an epidural was not on the table.

Nothing guarantees a pain-free birth. My mother had me by C-section under general anesthesia, and awoke while still intubated and opened up; the pain she felt for weeks after was tremendous. A good friend had her son by C-section with an epidural that wore off partway through. And the woman next to me in the postpartum ward after the birth of my first child had an epidural that worked fine for the delivery, but she spent the days afterward nearly incapacitated by pain. Even when all goes as it should with anesthetics, there comes a point when numbing ends and pain begins.

I didn't want to miss the birth of my child by being under anesthesia; besides, I'm horrible after being sedated. When I had my wisdom teeth out, I awoke thrashing and gagging, pulling the packing out of my mouth and stumbling around the recovery room. I wanted to be there and in my right mind when my kids were born, even if being there meant feeling everything. It wasn't masochistic, but I couldn't make myself believe that it wasn't painful. I try to keep an open mind, but when I hear women say that they experienced contractions as mere "rushes" of "intensity," or even as "ecstasy," I'm skeptical, and I think the vast history and prehistory of childbirth backs me up on this. It's telling that the very first pages of the

Bible offers an etiology of the phenomenon of pain in child-bearing. Why is there pain in childbirth? Certainly not because God wished it so, but only because of the fall, because of sin, because, as the story goes, human beings threw a wrench into paradise.

Pain in childbirth was for centuries addressed as a theological question, with certain (male) clergy throughout history insisting that any effort to alleviate pain in childbirth was an affront to God's wishes. In 1591, Agnes Sampson, a Scottish midwife suspected of witchcraft, was burned at the stake, apparently for trying to ease a woman's labor pangs with opium or laudanum. The nineteenth-century poet Julia Ward Howe (who's best remembered for the lyrics to "The Battle Hymn of the Republic") was deathly afraid of childbirth. Her own mother had died of puerperal fever ("childbed fever," as it was called) and Julia wanted to try chloroform, then just coming into vogue, to ease the pain of labor. Her husband, a famous medical doctor and philanthropist, dismissed her fears of dying in childbirth as evidence of her hypochondria and pooh-poohed the idea of using the pain relief that Queen Victoria, Julia's contemporary, gratefully accepted. "The pains of childbirth," wrote Dr. Howe, "are meant by a beneficent creator to be the means of leading [women] back to lives of temperance, exercise, and reason." I wonder what theological virtues Dr. Howe might have attributed to labor had he lived in a place where tradition called for a string to be tied around the father's testicles so that the mother could pull it with each contraction, thereby allowing both parents to share the pain.

In her 1970s bestseller, *Natural Childbirth and the Christian Family*, therapist Helen Wessel attempted to popularize, for an evangelical audience, the idea that pain in labor is a grotesque accretion of cultural myths, bad theology, and biblical misinterpretation. The Genesis story seems clear enough—*I will greatly increase your pains in childbearing,* God says to Eve. "I brought this problem up with Pastor Dirkson," says Carolyn, a fictional character in Wessel's didactic narrative. "He looked up the meaning of all the Hebrew and Greek words used about childbirth in the Bible, and discovered that there is nothing there that says women are meant to suffer pain when they bear a child. I want you and John to go ask him about this. He can explain it much better than I can."

It's telling that the fictional—and male—Pastor Dirkson's interpretation of the Greek and Hebrew, rather than Carolyn's previous childbirth experience, is what's meant to persuade the reader. "I've studied every passage," Pastor Dirkson says, "[and] checked the English translations against the original languages. [There's] not one single verse . . . that mentions any curse." In using the Bible—and male authority—to establish a rationale for natural childbirth, Wessel and others helped to create an evangelical and even patriarchal version of the natural childbirth movement that second-wave "difference" feminism launched. The feminist natural childbirth movement focused on reclaiming the goodness of womanhood and female bodies and their powerful ability to create and deliver life. Its reconsideration of the history of childbirth highlighted the relatively recent intrusion of male practitioners into what had, for millennia, been a womanly art, and one of the few somewhat respectable professions open to women of intelligence and learning—and therefore one that posed a challenge to the power and control of "medical men" and their instruments.

Wessel seems hopeful that the diabolical myth of pain in childbirth will be expunged; it's not to be found in the Hebrew and Christian Scriptures, she insists, but is rather a corruption introduced by Roman culture. "The Roman attitude toward the nuisance of childbearing and motherhood," she writes, "was in direct contrast to the continuing Jewish [and Christian] concept of the blessedness of marriage and children." If a woman does feel pain in childbirth, Wessel contends, its source is the woman's own psychological or physical tension—not the physiological process of birth itself. Which is to say, if you're in pain during labor, you have only yourself (and your possible ambivalence about motherhood) to blame—not Eve, not sin, not your husband, not God, not the evolution of big-brained bipedalism.

I understand Wessel's yearning for a world in which birth is joyful and painless—it's a longing for Eden, a vision of life flourishing and multiplying without the risk and pain to which fecundity is necessarily twinned. In Wessel's narratives, women never lack supportive partners, understanding clergy, adequate healthcare and housing, or anything else. That's nice for them, but this idealized vision of natural birth largely remains a privilege of white and relatively wealthy Western women, who, if they're being honest, will tell you that even with birthing tubs, birthing balls, doulas, heat packs, ice packs, meditation, and massage, bringing a baby into the world *hurts*. It hurts in the sort of way that puts one in mind of death. *I just remember thinking that I had to try and not die*, my friend Erika told me. *It was like being boiled alive in oil and not being able to die to get free of the pain*, thinks Katie Nolan in *A Tree Grows in Brooklyn*. Labor can be exhilarating, particularly at the beginning, when you think *is that all a contraction is?* That part passes, soon giving way to *no more* and *when will this end* and *help me*. I have never known anyone to deny it.

{An aside: the only generally representative and accurate portrayals of labor and childbirth I have seen on the screen are found in BBC's *Call the Midwife*. As is typical of people who have given birth or seen it done, my husband and I quit suspending our disbelief and start chuckling when Hollywood attempts to simulate human life's entry into the world. I can't quite figure this out. If Daniel Day-Lewis can plausibly represent anyone from Lincoln to a prizefighter, and Steven Spielberg can replicate the storming of the Normandy beaches so that veterans wept in recognition, and Pixar can create an animated film about the workings of an eleven year old's mind that entertains children and adults alike, why does nearly every movie and television birth have the production value of a so-so high school play? It's not as though human birth is an obscure phenomenon that's prohibitively cumbersome to research and document, like the mating dance of a bird-of-paradise.}

This is a total cliché, but it's also totally true: God and nature designed the pregnant body to reach a point where a woman is willing to do almost anything to get that baby out, even go through labor. Magazines for pregnant women always feature women who do not actually look pregnant but appear to have a tidily modified basketball tucked neatly into their yoga tops. *Where*, most pregnant women would ask, *are their hideously swollen feet? Why do they appear to be able to breathe through their noses, instead of gasping open-mouthed like most women in the third trimester?* Most actual pregnant women, toward the end, are a bit painful to look at. There's a definite sweet spot in most pregnancies where you look cutely rounded and resplendent with the Miracle of Life, but when the End is Nigh, even your nose looks pregnant and you can't wait to be alone in your body again.

American obstetricians and gynecologists do a lot of rushing to get the baby out, with high rates of medical induction of labor. My doctor in California openly admitted that this is often due to the fear of malpractice. *No doctor wants to be sitting in a courtroom with some lawyer saying, "Why, doctor, why didn't you do something?"* This was in the context of telling me that even though my baby seemed perfectly fine, she wanted me to check into the hospital that evening to evict the baby by pharmacological means. I'd already engaged in miles of waddling, eaten papaya and pineapple, and watched a feature-length murder mystery while attached to a wheezing, squeezing electric breast pump (a study I'd read suggested that this could be an effective means of induction). But nothing was working, and I was impatient, too, so I went along with the doctor's plan.

Tim and I went out to dinner and then to the hospital. I realized I had no camera—and this was before phones came equipped with them—so we picked up a few disposable ones on the way. We snapped a picture of ourselves together, smiling in the giant mirror in the hospital's birthing suite. I put on my hospital gown and folded my clothes fastidiously.

There's a picture of me, Virgin Mary–like in blue and white, one hand curled lovingly around my belly and the other holding a book—*The Secret Garden*. My hair is very long and shiny, and I've got my brand-new iPod earbuds in, listening to Yo-Yo Ma play Bach's unaccompanied cello suites. It is that calm before the storm, as beautiful and relaxed as *The Secret Garden*'s Collin, the malingering cousin of Mary Lennox, who strives for attention by pretending to be invalid. Mary revives him as she revives his mother's favorite walled garden, putting her hands in the dirt, clearing away weeds, watching things grow. He struggles to his feet; she struggles in the soil; both are reborn, but not without dirt, and not without tears.

A few minutes later, a nurse came in and administered something that, she said, was *just to get things ready to go*. Almost immediately, something was happening. Five minutes later, I said, *Um, this is actually hurting*. Ten minutes after that, the nurse came back in. She had been watching a screen in the nurses' station that measured the intensity of the contractions. *How we doing, honey?* She asked. I writhed and groaned and vomited into the trash can.

Six hours of darkness. I barely remember them. The nurse assigned to me had no idea how to help. Usually, she'd call for the anesthesiologist to administer the epidural he'd already told me I couldn't have, after squinting at my X-ray, tapping at my spine. *Um, breathe? That's it. Breathe all the way through?*

The nurse fled to watch my progress on the screen from her remote location and to call my doctor with periodic updates. So Tim and I crouched in that dim room, together and alone. My body was being wrenched apart in the middle by large, unseen hands. Once every few minutes the hands quit squeezing and twisting for ten seconds or so, and I would pant and beg for mercy until the hands resumed their determined effort. *Why does God want me to suffer?* I cried into Tim's chest. He held me, and his eyes brimmed too. Morning broke, and we watched it through the wide windows. Amazing that the cycle of evening and morning was still going on; for me, for us, there was only this moment, and this, now, now, *now*.

A new nurse arrived. *I used to assist at homebirths*, she said. *Let's get you off your back and onto this ball*, she said. In her presence, I suspected I was no longer stranded without a guide. A researcher walked in and asked to draw my blood for a research project. *You can say no,* the midwife whispered. I emitted a long and gravelly *no*. My body was mine right now.

There is a paradox in pregnancy in labor. While pregnant, one is the least alone one will ever be, embodying hospitality so radical that one functions as a house for another. Yet even though I had Tim, and then Tim *and* the kind nurse, I never felt so completely alone as I did when I gave birth to my first child. *I cannot pass this task to someone else. This is mine to bear, mine to bear; mine. I have to do this by myself. If I give up, if I do not drink this cup, they'll put me to sleep and take him out and I won't be there.* Jesus in Gethsemane, I think, would have been alone even if his friends had stayed, because some suffering cannot be shared. The philosopher Elaine Scarry suggests that the isolating nature of pain—the fact that it occurs within the perimeter of a single body and cannot actually be shared—means that physical torture is a particularly brutal form of solitary confinement—even the "unmaking" of a person's sense of his or her own existence. "Pain has an element of blank," Emily Dickinson wrote. "It cannot recollect / When it began, or if there were / A day when it was not."

This is what it takes to have a baby, this is what it takes to have a baby, the nurse whispered to me as I reached the point of breaking, and announced that I wanted to suspend the campaign. I thought, but did not say: *if this is what it is to have a baby, then I'm not sure I want one.* It was too late, of course, and to say such a thing would only have made me sound like a bad mother, or, in light of my Christian understanding of children as a blessing, ungrateful and maybe even rebellious against God's will. Jesus, sweating blood and begging for his suffering to be taken away, Jesus, dying and crying out because God had forsaken him: this is what I think of when I think of giving birth. Giving birth is what I think of when I think of Jesus' death. Here popular sentiments of "being in the moment" and "practicing gratitude" fail. Sometimes the present moment is hell, and your only song is lament.

Why did you choose to feel it all? I asked my friend Micha. We were floating in a backyard pool while her baby son napped in the shade nearby. She'd had a doula with her at his birth, two months earlier. *You could have gone through it without feeling anything, so why did you choose to feel pain?* Far more interesting than quasi-mythic tales of painless birth is this—in a culture that offers us the opportunity to avoid or alleviate nearly every kind of discomfort, why do some women choose to feel everything when they give birth? Why do they want to be there for some of the worst pain a body can live through?

A year earlier Micha and I floated in that same pool and talked about her recent painful miscarriage. *I felt like I needed to hurt, and even to bleed. As if my body needed to grieve too.* When she'd given birth several years earlier, with an epidural, she'd hated feeling that birth was something that happened *to* her instead of an event in which she was an active participant. How did it feel to have felt everything? Was she glad she had done it that way? She was. It had been a good, hard thing. I thought of another woman who chose to feel her second child's birth after her first child had died. *I wanted, I needed, to feel it all*, she said. So many women have named it as holy and profound: that redemptive movement from suffering to joy embodied in that most fundamental and bodily process of giving birth.

Among the prolific writings of the American preacher Cotton Mather (1663–1728) is a pamphlet, published in 1710 and splendidly titled *Elizabeth in Her Holy Retirement: An Essay to Prepare a Pious Woman for Her Lying-In, Or, Maxims and Methods of Piety to Direct and Support an Handmaid of the Lord Who Expects a Time of Travail*. In the twenty-first century, *Elizabeth in Her Holy Retirement* can easily be read as misogynistic and full of theological pronouncements that sound judgmental and scary. The very typeface is formidable; at one point, it changes to a brooding Gothic to adjure the pregnant woman: "Preparation for Death is that most Reasonable and Most Seasonable thing to which you must now Apply yourself."

Mather was a man acquainted with grief, and, for his time, forward thinking on modern medicine—specifically, vaccination. Three of his children, along with his wife, had died of measles, and though the method of inoculation Mather learned of from his enslaved servant, Onesimus, entailed a good deal of risk, Mather nonetheless preached that it was a good gift from God, and had his remaining children inoculated as Onesimus had been. He had a firebomb tossed through his window in response.

For Mather, pregnancy and childbirth are in essence *memento mori*: reminders that the woman—that we all—will one day die. But it would be unjust to accuse Mather of singling women out for especial haranguing. His sentiments are a far cry from Samuel Gridley Howe's insensitive dismissal of Julia's fears. Mather regards women's reproductive capacity as a spiritual boon. Why, he asks, are there more pious women than pious men, though roughly equal numbers of men and women are born? It is because women, exclusively, endure the pain and risk of childbirth, which, Mather says, "Make[s] you serious and cause[s] you seriously to consider on your condition, and bring you to a considerate, sollicitious [*sic*], Effectual preparation for Eternity." He is not reluctant to point out what women themselves surely knew: "You may have conceived That which determines but about Nine Month more at the most, for you to Live in the World." It's not that Mather is keen to see women die; rather, pastorally, he urges them to use the occasion of pregnancy to reflect on mortality, not so that they can make the adjustments necessary to avoid getting tossed into hell, but so that they, "being fit to Dy, . . . will be but the more fit to live." We moderns might be more inclined to embrace such insight when it comes from Buddhism or self-help literature than when it comes from eighteenth-century slave-holding Calvinists with unfortunate connections to a certain witch trial in Massachusetts, but Mather's is good wisdom still.

Those of us with access to Western hospitals don't need to feel pain, or not much, to give birth, and neither do we have to give much thought to mortality—though rates of maternal mortality in the United States, particularly among women of color, are unacceptably high. I wonder if our historically and globally unprecedented safety and comfort in childbirth—and germ theory and vaccinations and antibiotics and other life-saving innovations—have allowed many of the prosperous among us to forget that we, and our children, are still, finally, mortal. And I do wonder if those who choose to give birth without numbing, to voluntarily undergo a tremendously intense bodily experience, are something like extreme sports enthusiasts—ultramarathoners, obstacle racers, triathletes: seeking joyful confirmation within their bodies that, yes, they are here, they are truly alive. The difference is that we tend to applaud the athletes and accuse those who forgo pain medication of being martyrs. It's telling that in places and times that provide products and services to help us mostly avoid the pain and filth of life, the market also creates and commodifies dirty and painful experiences like Spartan Races and Tough Mudder, where middle-class people pay money and drive their SUVs to event sites so they can overcome painful and dirty obstacles. Is this a sign that some people are actually uncomfortable with their comfort? Does it indicate that joy, often enough, comes to us as we endure and transcend pain? Psychiatrist Viktor Frankl, whose wisdom was forged in suffering, warned against seeking after pain—"to suffer unnecessarily is masochistic rather than heroic"—but he also refused to equate it with powerlessness. Second-wave feminists Audre Lorde and Adrienne Rich spoke also about transforming pain into something usable; the latter noting that far from wanting to be rescued, many laboring women simply want to be guided; accompanied.

Just before noon, I closed my eyes, ignoring the orders barked by the nurse and doctor, arched my back, and bore down with an animal yell. I felt a river tumbling with raw potatoes rush through the bottom of my torso and between my legs. I opened my eyes to see a small, blue, kicking human in profile, dark hair and upturned nose sharp and distinct against the blood-spattered gown of the doctor holding him. Incredulous that my ordeal was over, I reached for him. I didn't forget my pain when I took him in my arms. I was holding him as the final contractions—the ones that deliver the placenta—rippled through me, and I cried out, *Why is it happening again?* The nurse, bless her, stayed past her shift to help me into the shower and a fresh nightgown while Tim cradled our son, and she whispered, *How do you feel now?* I felt invincible, mighty, godlike, intoxicated with love and ferociously protective of my baby. *He looks so familiar*, I said to everyone who would listen. *I recognize him.*

When we were newly married and still childless, Tim and I lived in the middle of a large wilderness area in Northern California. We'd see foxes and bears and even mountain lions from time to time; pretty much every week, we'd hike in the mountains. I learned to enjoy pushing a little further each time for the reward of a swim in a pristine mountain lake or a view of mountains beyond mountains beyond mountains. My favorite lake was framed by granite slopes reaching to the sky, the water on the far edge reaching for the horizon: endless, shining waters in the middle of a rocky place on the top of the world. We'd also kayak the river that ran through our mountains. Most of the rapids were safe and easily navigated; one was harmless but terrifying—they called it Hell's Hole; even skilled kayakers usually went under. There was a calm spot just before the hole where you could get out of the boat and onto the bank, walk past it, and get back into the water. Each time I kayaked the Trinity River, I forced myself to paddle over the edge, paddling hard to stay upright, always ultimately succumbing to the current. I'd tumble like a garment in a washer, and then the river would spit both me and my kayak back to the surface, where I would laugh maniacally. But each time I came to the edge, I'd be afraid. I'd have to talk myself into it all over again.

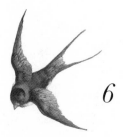

MOTHER

No human creature could receive or contain so vast a
flood of love and joy as I often felt after the birth of my
child. With this came the need to worship, to adore.

DOROTHY DAY, *THE LONG LONELINESS*

I have spent an inordinate amount of my life fearing the loss of those I love to the degree that I have in fact failed to love, to enjoy, to appreciate what I have had when I have had it. The lower animals, Wendell Berry suggests in one of his poems, do not tax their lives by fearing for the future, but I have been filing grief-ridden tax returns all my life, often only to realize that the burden of taxation has been levied largely by me.

Many people's first close encounter with death happens when a pet dies, and that's what happened to me. That the skinny gray kitten was sick was clear from the first day we brought him home from the shelter, but by that time I wouldn't think of returning him there. My mother and I brought him to a series of veterinarians, expecting an easy fix, but it turned out he had a feline immunodeficiency virus—*it's like AIDS in cats*, the vet explained—and was already quite sick. The shelter was very sorry; we could return the kitten, they said.

I wanted to keep him.

My dad sat on the edge of my bed as I cried. *He's going to die.*

He said that none of us knows what will happen in the future: *You might as well hold a healthy young kitten*, he said, *and cry because he's going to die* someday.

That was the problem, of course.

Most Christians believe in resurrection—at some point in the future, those who have died will follow in Jesus' footsteps and rise from the grave—but only some believe in what's called "the rapture." I was raised on this idea. Those who do believe it may happen at any time, and it will entail the sounding of a trumpet and the bodily appearance of Jesus on earth. Then, by a trick of levitation, faithful Christians will be beamed up to heaven, by way of the clouds. Not until adulthood did I realize that this doctrine conveniently furnishes its believers with the possibility of believing it possible to circumvent death and decay. As long as you believe that you might get to float up to heaven without passing through the morgue, you could trick yourself into imagining that the Grim Reaper might never actually come for you.

Most of the services my father officiated were memorial services rather than funerals, which is to say, there were no bodies in evidence. People in church, when I was very young, would often say that so-and-so "went to be with the Lord." I took this to indicate a more or less direct journey; a beam of holy light bathing the bed as the person began to rise, magically, miraculously, wafting through the ceiling and through the atmosphere, up into the invisible heavenly realms and Jesus' waiting arms. The way people talked at these funerals, it sounded like death was a good thing. "To live is Christ and to die is *gain*," or "Precious in the eyes of the Lord is the death of his saints," people would say. Neither Christian nor Jewish thought encourages a view of death as final and permanent, but that doesn't stop biblical writers from modeling lament.

For many of us, the process of dying and death is so remote from our experience—mediated and sanitized and cosmetically retouched by professionals—that we rarely have a chance to ponder its weightiness; its heaviness. We euphemize it with gentle phrases like "pass away." One Sunday morning in Malawi, my neighbor Belinda came by to walk me to the home of one of our students. She had given birth prematurely, and the baby had died. *The women have already prepared and buried the body this morning*, she said. This is the custom: the carpenter makes the coffin (never a casket, always a plain wooden box), and family and friends wash the body, place it in the coffin, carry the coffin, dig holes with shovels, and fill in the holes with dirt when they have placed the beloved one into the ground.

Belinda and I went into the woman's house and sat on the floor with her and her mother and sister. This was an expected, ritualized visit, like sitting shiva in Jewish families. There is no bulletin, no sermon, no set-apart space, no clerical intercession, nothing except people sitting on the ground together, mostly silently.

If that sick shelter kitten introduced me to the apparently irrevocable loss death represents—because apart from the hope that the resurrection will be general enough to include every dead creature, what is death but irrevocable loss?—it induced in me an urgency in prayer and a determination to nurture. I fed the cat with a spoon. I prayed for him. In the end, the vet came to take him away to euthanize him, and returned him, frozen solid, in a black garbage bag. My dad buried it without any of us looking at the cat again.

The humorist Mallory Ortberg has said that prayers like "fix this" and "fix me" don't work. The only prayer that works, she says, is "'hi'—which is really a way of saying 'abide with me.'" I still regret sending that poor little shelter cat off to "pass away," instead of abiding with him until the end.

A neighbor in Malawi came by with a puppy in a shoebox, and the boys fell in love. We wanted a dog to protect the boys from snakes as they played in the yard and to discourage would-be intruders, including the monkeys and baboons who regularly pilfered from the vegetable gardens. Aidan named the puppy Little Ann after the female hound in *Where the Red Fern Grows*, one of the many children's classics that involves the death of a dog. Our Little Ann died, too, and quickly, of parvovirus, which kills even puppies lucky enough to land in a Western veterinary hospital. Tim and I did our best, holding her, dripping fluids in her mouth, administering the medicine we'd scrounged. *Let's just let her lie down*, we agreed. She exhaled once and died with a rush of blood and water.

James, our housekeeper, came, and his shoulders dropped when he saw. He cleaned up the mess. *Keep the body here for the moment*, I asked.

Let's ask the boys if they want to see her, Tim and I agreed, *but they don't need to see the blood.*

We have sad news, we said.

My son cried himself to sleep in my lap, though it was the middle of the day. When he awoke, he and Tim built a little house out of LEGOs and surrounded it with a garden. *Let's put in lots of trees and flowers.*

James carried the little body to the back yard in a cardboard box, and dug a hole and buried her in the garden, where he would plant the maize—the staple crop in Malawi—a few weeks later.

My son never wanted to read another story in which the dog dies, and I never wanted another dog. But there were still snakes in the yard and thieving monkeys and rats, too, and we needed a dog. So, a few months later we bought a little German shepherd pup from a breeder in town, and I bleached everything that could be bleached to clean the parvovirus, and I vaccinated the dog against parvo myself, after watching a tutorial online. I cooked special food. I was unsentimental. I just didn't want another little grave in the garden.

I wrote a story about my doomed shelter cat, and read it aloud to my story group—a circle of five American expats in St. Andrews, Scotland. We met twice monthly to read our personal narratives—written on a common theme—aloud. My son was very young then, and I was rushed and slapdash, sketching out stories on the backs of Tim's academic papers in between nap time and mealtime and bedtime. What I read to the four women was humorous, mock heroic, as if I, a child, was merely pretending to serious emotion, serious action. But my friend Nicole, a priest and a doula, wouldn't dismiss it as such. *It's not a story about pretending. It's a story about mothering.* That seemed true. It was a story in which I tried everything—feeding, holding, praying—to hold on to a mortal creature that I had lost.

That is what it is to be a mother: to love and nurture that which is fragile, mortal, unpredictable, uncontrollable, and ultimately not even truly one's own. Kathleen Norris put it this way: "One of the most astonishing and precious things about motherhood is the brave way in which women consent to give birth to creatures who will one day die."

Solomon, the king of Israel, prayed for wisdom, and he prayed for it as a parent might pray, as the harried mother of multiple small children might pray—*I am your servant in the midst of people so numerous they cannot be counted. Give me an understanding heart.* An unselfish prayer, which God was pleased to answer—*I have given you a wise and understanding*

heart. And the first tale of Solomon's wisdom defines the essence of mother love—and of God's love.

Two mothers stand before the king with but one living baby between them. "The living child is mine and the dead one is yours," each says. "Bring a sword," Solomon says. "Divide the living child in two. Give half to one and half to the other." The woman who had deceived the other by exchanging her own dead child for the living child agrees: let it be neither yours nor mine. Divide it.

She is a woman with nothing to lose.

I pity this woman, this grieving woman, but the story is less about her grief than about the nature of mother love in its ideal form; love that forfeits control, protection, and even justice for the sake of life. "O my lord, give her the living child," the true mother says, so identifying herself to Solomon and to any discerning heart.

How do you discern a mother? Look for the person who relinquishes her claim to being right for the sake of life.

I was a student at a strictly patriarchal Bible college when someone handed me Phyllis Trible's *God and the Rhetoric of Sexuality*, which among other things explores the Bible's use of feminine language in describing God. Trible identifies the love that the Bible associates with wombs as love that "protects and nourishes but does not possess and control." The womb—*rehem*—is, she suggests, regarded as the seat of compassion—*rahamim*. "To the responsive imagination, this metaphor suggests the meaning of love as selfless," Trible writes. Throughout the Hebrew Bible, "the divine and the maternal intertwine. . . . In biblical traditions, an organ unique to the female becomes a vehicle pointing to the compassion of God."

In the middle of the night, more than a decade ago, I cuddled my newborn son, my firstborn, against my shoulder, breathing in his baby smell, memorizing the gentle motion of his tiny ribcage rising and falling, almost imperceptibly. The time in which he would fit comfortable in one arm would be so short, I knew; soon he would struggle out of my arms. Soon enough he would run from me, would be embarrassed to be kissed by me, would no longer want to hold hands in a crowd, but not to let him go—to withhold his freedom—would be to fail in my most fundamental maternal task. I held him close, inhaling him—*this is now, this is now, this is now.* I felt enmeshed in, and almost strangled by, love for him.

This is the pain of love: to open one's heart to loss, to rejection; to cede control.

This is the pain of God's love: when the people to whom God gave birth forget the Rock that begot them. When they forget their mother.

I grew out of playing with animals paired two-by-two and realized that the story about Noah and his ark and the flood was not about lovable zoo creatures going for a cruise but was in fact a story of massive human destruction. *How could a loving God . . . ?* None of the answers satisfy: *what you should be noticing,* I've heard it said, *is that God saved anyone at all.* This, I think, is of little comfort in the face of all that death—when the picture of God offered for our consideration is a picture that terrifies: a parent drowning her own children. Why create them, only to destroy them?

How unimaginably awful do things have to be for a parent to cry out for the death of a child? When a cholera epidemic rippled through Cincinnati, Ohio, in 1849, Harriet Beecher Stowe's youngest child, her admitted favorite, just four years old, suffered dreadfully and died. Cholera is a particularly nasty way to go; daily you lose several gallons of fluid out of your body through violent, uncontrollable diarrhea, and you may turn wrinkly and blue and suffer seizures before it is over. Stowe wrote in a letter:

My Charley—my beautiful, loving baby, so sweet, so full of life and hope and strength—now lies shrouded, pale and cold, in the room below. . . . I have just seen him in his death agony, looked on his imploring face when I could not help nor soothe nor do one thing, not one, to mitigate his cruel suffering, do nothing but pray in my anguish that he might die soon.

If it seems a great evil, inconceivable, really, for a mother to long for her child to die, consider how great the besetting evil must be. An imperfect analogy. Still.

God grieved at the violence and wickedness of humankind upon the earth. Each imagination of the thoughts of their hearts was only evil continually, and it grieved God's heart that God had made them. Pause here, and empathize with this maternal God—God grieved the very existence of the beings made in her own image, for her own delight. So violent, so evil had these beings become that to obliterate the masterpiece and crown of the creation seemed the lesser evil. It is easy to think this cruel, but when we consider the evil and the violence and the corruption in this world, say, the Third Reich's diabolically efficient killing machine, and ask why God didn't do something to stop it, what, exactly, do we have in mind?

The flood story is a story of starting again. Abort, retry, fail? The narrative does not encourage the reader to picture the choking and drowning of all life, presumably, of children and elderly along with women and men. Rather the flood story unfurls like a film played in reverse, where all that is folds back into all that wasn't; where all that is becomes as it was before. Once again, all is formless and void, and God's Spirit hovers like a dove, that symbol of peace, over the surface of deep water. Erasing the memory of violence, of evil, a grieving God washes away the beloved, the beautiful creation, to begin it again. God washes it with water, with a flood, giving grace in the buoyancy of the ark and grace in the obliterating depths of the waters of destruction and renewal, waters rippled by God's tears.

Scholars say that every civilization has and must have its flood story, and that the one in Genesis is simply Israel's: it is only a question, they say, of how to make sense of the flood story within the larger story of the goodness of creation and the presence of the Creator who endowed people with reason and with freedom: reason and freedom that they spent on wickedness and great evil. For God to stem the thoughts of people's hearts from only evil continually would be to rescind their freedom. A love that nourishes and protects, but does not control: a maternal love does not rescind freedom, does not preclude the possibility of forgiveness, of a clean start. The waters cover the wickedness; enveloping the world back into the womb of God to be born again.

Why couldn't God just? . . . I don't know the question, much less the answer.

I am still not quite satisfied with this story. I am trying to see in it a story of freedom and of the cost of freedom, a story of the risk we run in love and the risk God runs in loving, a story of the buoyancy of grace, a story that ends with the dove, that old symbol of the Holy Spirit and of peace, spreading gentle wings over the waters, olive branch in her beak, God hovering above the primordial waters once again to separate light from dark, water from land, night from day.

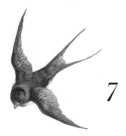

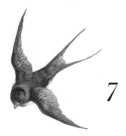

7

BAPTIZE

transitive verb

1 religion: to administer baptism

*2 a : to purify or cleanse spiritually, especially
by a purging experience or ordeal*

b: initiate

Women tell birth stories. People celebrate birthdays, as do nations. The people of God, the Israelites, have several birth stories, several birth days, but the most definitive, the one God insists on their celebrating, is the exodus—the mass exodus, the deliverance, the emergence of the people of Israel from slavery in Egypt, observed annually as Passover. "We were slaves, now we're free, let's eat," my mother's cousin Joe would say, nodding to the religious significance of the occasion before digging into beef brisket and noodle kugel. By contrast, with my parents and our profoundly hospitable Orthodox Jewish friends, including a rabbi, we observed an elaborate, ritualized retelling of the birth story of my mother's people, of my people; the story in which God, the midwife, liberates suffering slaves from their bondage in *mitsrayim*—the Hebrew word for Egypt, which, as it happens, is related to the word for the pain of labor contractions.

Birth itself induces Pharaoh's hate and desire for domination when he notices that the Israelites in his land exceed Egyptians in number and power: their fertility is threatening. Yet in the upside-down logic of so many biblical narratives— *the last shall be first, blessed are the poor, when I am weak then I am strong*—increasingly ruthless Egyptian opposition only escalates Israel's expansion. Pharaoh revises his plans, directing his efforts at the fountainhead of Israelite abundance— their apparently astonishing fecundity, and the custodians of that fruitfulness: the midwives. *Kill every baby boy while the mother is yet on the birthstool. Collapse the moment of birth and the moment of death into one.*

Well before Moses grudgingly agrees to be God's assistant midwife in bringing Israel out of the protracted labor of their bondage, the midwives Shiphrah and Puah embody the courage and integrity that every midwifery manual I've ever come across—ancient, medieval, modern—cites as requirements of the profession. I imagine them with strong hands and a calm and cheerful demeanor, past childbearing age themselves, knowing eyes sparkling in sun-crinkled faces. Surely they knew that to defy the Pharaoh was to risk their own lives, but defy him they did, risk be damned. Their explanation, their honorable lie, is just what I would expect from a midwife: a nonchalant, self-effacing and possibly feminist pronouncement on their clients' knack for giving birth speedily and easily. *Hebrew women are so vigorous they hardly need us; the babies are out by the time we can get there.* These unshrinking women are the midwives not just for individual Hebrew women. They are the midwives of the nation of Israel, uncomplicated both in their ardent commitment to the preservation of life that defines their profession and in their fear of God.

Frankly, Shiphrah and Puah make Moses look pretty puny.

Very well, Pharaoh says. *You can't conflate the moment of birth with the moment of death? Throw the boys in the Nile, then. Transform that water, that source of life and fertility, into a burial ground.* Then, of course, there is the brave mother hiding her baby boy in a vessel she fashions to shelter him: a basket—a little ark—of papyrus and bitumen and pitch. She casts it among the reeds at the bank of the Nile, while his sister, perhaps his sister Miriam, brave soul, watches, waits, and arranges for her own mother, for the baby boy's own mother, to nurse him for wages until such time as the Pharaoh's daughter could raise him as her own, naming him Moses because *I drew him out of the water.*

From the water of his possible death, his second mother draws him out: a second birth.

This story appears at the beginning of the book of Exodus and also encapsulates it. The story of God's deliverance of Israel is a birth story: God, the midwife, God, the mother, vigorously bearing Israel through Egypt, *mitsrayim*, labor pains, tunneling through the sea that could so easily overcome them, delivering them to dry land. "Narrow was the passageway through the Red Sea and narrow is the birth canal that stretches to allow the child out," as Tikva Frymer-Kensky puts it in her book of prayers and blessings for pregnant women, making explicit the suggestion that the passage through the Red Sea can be envisioned as a passage through a symbolic birth canal. And Miriam, Moses's sister, rejoices when they are delivered.

Take note: the people echoing God's deliverance, in this précis, this pithy preview, are women. They are midwives and mothers of a nation: matriarchs. They are the hands and feet and images of God, a mother God, a midwife God, braving suffering, moving strongly through the risk of death to the promise of life; of fruitful, flourishing life.

Tim and I have lived in four different countries on three different continents and in three different US states since our two sons were born, in 2005 and 2008. Aware of our peregrinations, people are often curious to hear my children talk about their travels—and not infrequently about their respective birthplaces. Aidan, our firstborn, was the fifth- or sixth-generation male Stone to be born in Shasta County, California, but Graeme was born in Scotland, and has a Scottish birth certificate.

When asked, "Where were you born?" Graeme has sometimes replied, "In a bathtub." He pretends not to know what's really meant by the question, and enjoys the laugh that this elicits.

The birth pool at Forth Park Maternity Hospital in Kirkcaldy was less like a bathtub and more like the baptistery in the church in Greenport where I grew up. I pitied those poor paedobaptists (as we Baptists referred to them) who merely sprinkled water from fonts onto babies who wouldn't even remember. Our baptisms were much more dramatic, usually involving adults telling exciting conversion stories in which the person about to be baptized recounted all sorts of thrilling but ultimately unfulfilling sins of which he or she had now repented before being immersed by my dad. Our baptistery was made for full-body dunking.

The baptistery was under the floor where my father stood to preach on ordinary Sundays, an arrangement not dissimilar from that for the Bedford Falls High school gymnasium in *It's a Wonderful Life*, into which Jimmy Stewart and Donna Reed plunge unexpectedly while dancing the Charleston, all while misapprehending the shrieking of the crowd as approbation of their performance. The floor beneath the pulpit was flimsy. During a boring sermon I amused myself by it giving way as in a dunk-the-clown carnival gag, accidentally rebaptizing my very surprised dad. I used to help him fill it, and sometimes longed to take a dip in it myself, after I'd learned to swim, but though we Baptists didn't believe in such a thing as holy water, to swim in a baptistery would've constituted some kind of sacrilege nonetheless.

I arrived at the hospital in Scotland laboring hard, contractions coming so close together that it took considerable time simply to move from the car to the front door. Sitting in the car, I breathed and hummed through one contraction, then got out of the car, walked several feet, and stopped to breathe and hum through another. I repeated this process several times, entered, repeated it several more, and finally made it to the midwifery unit. "Ach, but you're just a wee lass! We're gonna hafta let some water out o' the bearth pool!" The midwife greeted me cheerfully and led me into the assigned room where, in the shamelessness of labor, I stripped to the skin piece by piece, strewing my clothes about and staggering toward the pool. I lowered myself into the calm water of the rectangular birth pool so very like the baptistery of my Baptist childhood.

It is one thing to say that Jesus is the bread of life, and another to put the bread the priest has consecrated and declared to be the body of Christ into your mouth and chew it. It is one thing to talk about the symbolism of water, so suggestive of both life and death, and to imagine grace and alleviation as a buoy and hope as an anchor through turbulent and painful times—and it is another to rock back and forth, creating literal ripples and swells that slosh and slap with the rhythm of your own body's rumbling; with the movement that comes both from you and through you, that is you and is not you, the child within you struggling to move through the waters of your womb, the you that cries out, both captain and captive on this voyage, both dependent upon and grateful for the comfort offered by your traveling companions, yet aware also of being so nearly alone inside your skin.

I rocked and moaned, and as the time grew very near, cried out, or, more precisely, bellowed. When each swell subsided, I whispered apologies, conscious still of my surroundings, and not wanting to be perceived as the "loud American" of British stereotypes. *Don't apologize, you brave lass, you're doing so well!* In childbirth, what appears to be weakness—hollering, for example—is simply the steam being given off by fiery strength.

Christians use the image of God as a warrior much more than they consider the image of God as a laboring woman. Whether they are looking to God as warrior as justification for wars (cultural or otherwise) or with an amalgam of discomfort and confusion, as in historic peace-church traditions and certain progressive and mainline churches, it is not an unfamiliar image. But Christians across the spectrum of cultural, theological, and political points of view seem equally to neglect biblical images of God as a laboring woman.

These images seem relatively few when compared to the image of God as warrior; perhaps that explains the discrepancy, though I suspect a different cause: one deeply rooted in shame about women's bodies, vestigial theological misunderstandings about the nature of pain in childbirth (that is, believing that it is a curse) and the pervading sense that God, who is spirit, is somehow, in fact, more like a man, a *man's* man, than like a woman.

God as warrior doesn't do much for me, but I cherish the image of God as a laboring woman. The book of Isaiah joins the two images closely enough that I can imagine they share more in common than I might have suspected: the Lord goes forth like a warrior, stirring up fury, crying out, shouting, and showing himself mighty—and, in the next line, switches to the first person to speak as a laboring woman: *I will cry out like a woman in labor, I will gasp and pant.* Here God is a woman warrior, preparing to create something new. She is the creator of all that has come before, and, in the crisis and agony of labor, everything seems to be coming apart, undone, like the de-creation of the flood. She will level rough places, she will dry up the lakes, she will turn rivers into islands. This entails suffering, struggling, panting, bellowing: but she is making something new. Her pain is not destructive, it is not meaningless, it is productive. It is fruitful. It begets new life for the children she has begotten and will continue to beget:

Do not fear. I have redeemed you. I will call you by name. You are mine. When you pass through the waters, I will be with you. When you pass through the rivers, they shall not overwhelm you. When you walk through the fire, you will not be burned.

I was passing through those waters, through those rivers, and the fire had begun to burn, unquenched even by the waters.

No more! I moaned. *God, please, no more.*

You will meet your baby very soon, the midwife whispered. I held Tim's arms, which, just above the surface of the water, held me. A student midwife, quietly observing from the corner, mouthed her encouragement—*almost there!* Then he was there, this stranger, passing through the waters of my womb and the waters of the birthing pool, drawn out of the waters with my own hands. I gazed at his red, swollen face that, even with its squashed nose, looked, as had his brother's, strangely familiar. *It's you, of course. Here you are.* He squalled at the indignity and discomfort of his journey.

"Hello, Graeme," Tim said.

Hello, Graeme. I said.

Do not fear. I have delivered you. I have called you by name, and you are mine. You have passed through those waters, and I was with you, and I am with you, and I will be with you.

You cannot convince me that the birth pool was not in fact a baptistery, that the water from which he was taken was not holy water, that I, his mother, was not, by God's help, godlike in my deliverance, in guiding him through the waters of my womb, through the waters of his first baptism, that perilous voyage through the sea, and calling him by name.

In Judaism, a woman immerses herself in the *mikveh*—the ritual bath—after she gives birth, not because she is dirty, but because in giving life it is as if she has touched death.

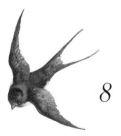

VESSEL

From the very beginning down to the latest stages of development we find this archetypal symbol as essence of the feminine. The basic symbolic equation woman = body = vessel corresponds to what is perhaps mankind's—man's as well as woman's—most elementary experience of the Feminine.

ERICH NEUMANN, *THE GREAT MOTHER*

I had two toy potter's wheels when I was young, both plastic. One was hospital-bed almond; the other several complementary primary colors, but neither was sturdy enough to do much more than frustrate me to the point of giving up. I might have made something from the air-drying clay, but more likely I was as sparing with it as I almost always was with art and craft supplies, saving it for some future masterpiece I was sure to make, only to leave it so long that it dried out completely and became unworkable.

My itch to fashion things from clay never abated, and when I found myself at the Play-Doh table with my toddler son, mindlessly sculpting what turned out to be a very convincing pig, I gave some thought to trying pottery again. Several years later, I found myself in a ceramics studio on the shore of Lake Malawi, which is so vast that it feels like an inlet or bay, though the water is fresh and shallow for many yards.

"Make sure to bring bathing suits and snorkels, because Lake Malawi is gorgeous," a fellow missionary advised us as we were packing to move. Others—including our doctor and more than a few guidebooks—warned against swimming in the lake because of the risk of bilharzia (also called schistosomiasis), a kind of flatworm parasite that lives in, and is released by, freshwater snails. The larvae penetrate the skin of the swimmers and bathers and fishermen and women scrubbing laundry and kids playing at the water's edge, then migrate to the urinary tract to feed off the blood supply there and to reproduce indefinitely. Schisto infections are common enough in sub-Saharan Africa that some—perhaps many— communities don't realize that the normal color of pee isn't pink. And though the World Health Organization considers it second only to malaria as the world's most economically devastating disease, schisto doesn't have particularly effective PR, which is particularly unfortunate since the infection seems to make its sufferers even more susceptible to infection with HIV.

"You just take a couple of pills four to six weeks after you've been in the lake, and you're fine," seemed to be the expat consensus. It's true enough: schisto is usually treatable with a dose or two for about twenty-five cents, making it yet another of those diseases that NGO workers and travelers and missionaries have to be aware of but probably not too alarmed over, even as those very same diseases—malaria and rabies, for example—regularly create orphans and obligate women to bury their children and grandchildren. And it's one of those things that from the vantage point of the privileged West seems like it'd be no trouble to fix—sell some recycled paper bead necklaces or pass the donation basket. It isn't that more money and awareness wouldn't help. It would. But even cheap and simply fixed—things that might work well in one small village—don't always scale up well, for a thousand million quirky little reasons that are hard or impossible to guess.

Insecticide-treated bed nets, for example are—or once were—considered one of the best defenses against malaria. They're cheap and effective, and Westerners like contributing money to purchase them. As we bumped along the road to Lake Malawi, though, deeper and deeper into the rural places where most of the population dwells, I noticed mosquito netting inexpertly covering the window openings. Later, on the shores of the lake itself, I saw groups of men holding the edges of enormous nets, bringing in a meager catch. It was not a fishing net, however, but an enormous nine-patch of bed nets of different sizes and colors, sewn together. This is about as good for the health of the lake and the fish and the Malawians as you might expect, but getting malaria is an abstract concern in the face of hunger. Anxiety over infectious disease—like most anxiety, as I'm painfully aware—is a mark of privilege. It is a luxury that can only be indulged when the fear of hunger ("the only fear," according to some sub-Saharan African proverbs) has been more or less vanquished.

We arrived at the lake after seven dusty hours in our rusted and rattling Land Rover; the rubber soles melted off my sandals. I was furiously hot. Wordlessly, I flapped down to the lake's edge and waded up to my neck, entirely clothed; partially shod. Graeme followed suit; Aidan, the first-born rule follower, stood on shore, regarding our recklessness. I can still feel the relief of the water freeing the dust from my skin, diluting salt from my scalp, cooling my very soul. I left the water as a new person, dripping, laughing, and, laying aside the microbial situation, clean.

The pottery lodge drew people just for the location—simple cabins facing a white-sand beach and the teal of Lake Malawi; Mozambique a thin black strip on the far horizon on a clear day. On most days, you see fishermen in dugout canoes with carved paddles, and from certain vantage points, you could be forgiven for forgetting what century you were in. Women carried baskets handwoven from dried grasses; a young man drove a herd of skinny cattle along the water's edge. We could watch it all from the simple, open studio, where we had come on a learning vacation, ready to study the ancient craft of making earthen vessels.

To watch an experienced potter lift a tall, graceful bowl or vase from a large gray lump is to watch a conjuring of sorts; form given to that which was formless, someone's idea given shape, transformed into something that could hold water and flowers, or stew and rice. The spinning wheel reveals the clay's essential liquidity; nudged this way or that, it gives and flows, ripples and spreads. It's an elegant process, beautiful as ballet, but when I sat down at the wheel to give it a whirl, I felt like a hippo in a tutu.

We had signed up for a three-week ceramics course, which included instruction in traditional Malawian pottery, taught by two women from the village: one Anglican, one Muslim, named Gloria and Fatima, respectively. Traditional Malawian pottery is slow and meditative compared to the electric whirl of the modern wheel, and I soon found that it appealed to me much more than the wheels that I'd always longed to get my hands on. Fatima and Gloria spoke almost no English, and I spoke almost no Chichewa, so they taught me as one teaches the very old or the very young: a nod and a smile of approval, or else a shake of the head and a gentle redirection; a nudge of the hand here to indicate how my finger should curve, a hand placed over mine to mold it into the right position for shaping a rim.

Traditional pots start with a lump of rough, red clay that's gathered, Gloria and Fatima managed to tell me, from termite mounds, which is putting it delicately: it's termite poop. Every pot, no matter the size, starts with about as much clay as you can comfortably hold in one hand. You hold it in one palm and slap it with the other, turn it, and slap it again, until you have a dense, squat cylinder of sorts, which you nest into a small, rounded base—something like the remnants of a broken bowl. With one palm holding the clay steady, you use two fingers of one hand to make a small indentation in the middle of the cylinder. Push down, pull up, rotate the cylinder; push down, pull up, rotate and repeat. It's slow, and the clay is rough with sand and tiny pebbles, which sometimes must be picked out and flicked away. But it's okay if you pull too hard and make a hole; this clay is forgiving and cracks are easily repaired. You take a shell from the beach and use it to flare the sides of the pot and to turn a fluted rim. You give it shape, and then you give it time in the sun to dry part way. Later, you scrape it from the base pottery and polish the new pot with a smooth stone until it's shiny. You wouldn't think that pebbly termite poop could be made into something shiny and sturdy with your two hands, some broken pottery, and a pebble, but there it is. Scratch some designs into the clay if you like, or leave it plain. Build a fire around the pots with the dried out sticks of a cassava plants and piles of dry grass, let it burn; let it ash over. When all has cooled, you pull out the pots and clean them. There they are, black and red, smooth, shiny, and whole.

Judith and Yusuf, both Malawians trained in European-style ceramics, were our main teachers on the course, and through them I asked Gloria and Fatima to teach me Chichewa as we went along, seated on the clay tile floor, slowly turning termite poop into beautiful, useful pottery. The wide, shallow pot that curved in and then flared out at the top was an *mpica,* used for cooking and serving *ndiwo,* the vegetable stew or "relish" that daily adds flavor and nutrition to the cornmeal mush—*nsima*—which is the staff of life for most Malawians. Could they teach me to make a big pot? I asked and gestured—could I make a *huge* one? A few more *mpica,* for practice; then, they said, I'd be ready to attempt an *msugo.*

"Gloria," I asked. "Teach me how to say that I don't want any bananas." Judith translated, and Gloria laughed.

"*Ine sindikufuna masamba, ayi!*" she said. I repeated this, and she laughed again.

"*Masamba*," she said, and shaped her hands around an imaginary banana.

"*Ine*," she said, pointing to herself.

"*Sin-dikufuna*," she said, emphasizing the first word and shaking her head so as to indicate "no."

"*Ine sindikufuna madzi, ayi!*" she said, pushing away a water glass and indicating with her facial expression that she didn't want it.

"*Ine dikufuna* Coca-Cola, *basi*," she said, cackling with laughter.

I *don't* want water, *no*. I want Coca-Cola, *only*. I don't want bananas, *no*. I want mangos, only. I repeated the lines, varying the nouns, pointing to objects to find out the names, piecing together sentences from scraps of Chichewa I overheard and looked up in my tattered dictionary, copying Gloria's phrases and her accent and her gestures until both of us were laughing hard. Malawians talk with their hands and faces, Gloria said somehow, and I somehow understood. In these exchanges I was the happiest and most connected I'd ever been in Malawi. The cliché "ships passing in the night" is often aptly applied to crosscultural communication, even when language is not a barrier, a barrier I bumped against daily in the Malawian city of Zomba, where we lived. It's a kind of magic, I decided, when, despite lacking a shared language, you manage to laugh with and learn from another human being, however imperfectly, however faltering the attempt.

As I grew more comfortable with Gloria and Fatima, I broke one of the traveler's rules for eating in developing countries, where parasites are rampant, and ate with my hands out of a common bowl. Each morning at the pottery lodge, at ten o'clock, we paused for a tea break. Gloria and Fatima cooked rice or *batatas*—sweet potatoes—over charcoal outside, and the staff and the students sat around the table, passing sugar and milk, shyly and awkwardly the first few times, and increasingly rowdy thereafter. Gloria, Fatima, Judith, and sometimes Yusuf would reach into the bowl of roasted *batatas* and, pulling off a piece, pop it into their mouths. *Batata*, Gloria said, pointing. *Zikomo, ine dikufuna batata*, I said. *Please, I want a sweet potato.* Gloria grinned her wide grin that was almost a grimace and handed me the bowl.

Nearly every act of eating and drinking in Malawi was preceded by strategic harm reduction acts: I washed vegetables in a bleach solution, peeled what could be peeled, cooked what could be cooked, and filtered all water—even that used for toothbrushing—through a trio of Swiss-made ceramic cylinders capable of intercepting even the minutest microbes. Partaking of the Eucharist at church was a challenge: one would rather not be fearing one's neighbor's germs when sharing the bread and wine that are supposed to be the outward sign of spiritual unity among the community of the baptized, but I couldn't quite manage not to wonder how well-scrubbed the priest's hands were when he put the wafer on my tongue, and I was never able to not wince inwardly when I sipped wine from the common cup.

So when Gloria handed me the bowl of sweet potatoes, and showed me how she pinched off a portion, peel and all, and ate it, smiling, I followed suit. Its skin was taut and crisp, the flesh butter-smooth and creamy, lightly sweet with a hint of smokiness from being cooked over coals. There was no comparison between the *batata* and the artificially flavored tea biscuits that usually appeared on the tea table, and I enjoyed this companionable light meal, ignoring, for the moment, the risks and the warnings against eating food from less-than-pristine sources. For that moment, at least, I was willing to risk whatever may have come from sharing a common bowl, and that, too, felt like a little bit of magic; a tiny crack of light.

I thought a lot about biblical metaphors involving pottery and clay while I was taking the pottery course. The Creator God is envisioned as a ceramicist in the Genesis narratives—the verb for *form*, as in "the Lord God *formed* a human from the dust of the ground" is related to the words used to describe a potter's craft. Throughout the Hebrew Bible and New Testament, writers describe the human condition in terms of pottery and clay. Human beings are earthen *vessels*, made from the same stuff as dirt yet containing within them the very breath of God; fashioned from something that comes from the ground, yet made in God's own image. Conceiving of human beings as pottery emphasizes the humility of the materials and the artisan's skill; implying, at least, for the writer in Job, that the potter—in this case, God—has an abiding affection and concern for the pieces she has crafted: "Remember that you fashioned me like clay, / and will you turn me to dust again?" (Job 10:8-9). The book of Isaiah—which imagines God as birthing mother and midwife more than any other biblical book—also invokes images of clay, pottery, and artisans repeatedly, both to emphasize the humility humans should have before the divine maker, as well as to express the affection implied in that relationship: "We are all the work of your hand" (Isaiah 64:8).

What I thought about most often as I sat with Gloria and Fatima, making pots by hand from the rough, red termite clay, were the passages in the New Testament that speak of some pots being made for ceremonial use, while others are made for humble, ordinary use. It is not for us to question the potter as to why—all pots, whether plain or fancy, come from the same source and share the same essential qualities that make them what they are. So too do all humans, whether paupers or princes, whether educated or ignorant, come from women's wombs. *There is a loveliness about even the simplest pot*, I found myself thinking. *And it takes the same level of skill to make a fancy pot as to make a humble one—if both are to function as they should. If they are to hold water.*

I thought a lot about the pot as an image not just of human beings in general but of women in particular; I'd been reading the poet Adrienne Rich's classic feminist book *Of Women Born: Motherhood as Experience and Institution*, which braids history, philosophy, memoir, and literature in exploring "the power and powerlessness embodied in motherhood." What looks like powerlessness in motherhood is often powerful—the woman straining and crying out and losing control of bowel and bladder as she pushes her baby into the world appears weak at the moment that is, in fact, the peak of her strength. Anthropologists, Rich notes, talk about how, in many cultures, pottery-making was invented and practiced by women, exclusively, and was in some cases as off-limits to men as the practice of midwifery. Thinking about women in connection with containers is uncomfortable, Rich acknowledges, since it reinforces the notion that women, as sexual beings and mothers, are merely passive and receptive—*receptacles*.

But it's not that simple: even if, as Rich suggests, a woman potter "molded, not simply vessels, but images of herself, the vessel of life, the transformer of blood into life and milk," this image is not one that lacks power but embodies it: "the vessel is anything but a passive receptacle; it is transformative, active, powerful," turning milk into yogurt and cheese, transforming pressed grapes into wine, grain into beer, and ash and fat into soap. Pottery takes the stuff of the ground and transforms it into something that is itself transformative. Pottery gives birth to culture, in every sense.

I wore shame like a scarf in Malawi, always draped around my shoulders, brushing the back of my neck, rendering me flushed and uncomfortable. I could easily spend on a single restaurant meal what a domestic worker—a *fortunate* worker—might earn in a month. Even our simplest meals at home were far better than what most Malawians eat on most days. It pains me to admit that even our dog ate better than many people. Our clothes and shoes, our education, our money, our access to medical care, and, above all, the fact that we always had options available to us, including the option to pack up and leave—well, all of it overwhelmed me, particularly at home, in the city of Zomba where we lived, where I was supposed to be teaching a language I felt bad my students had to learn.

I was afraid, and still am, that everything I did in Malawi was all wrong, that, despite my best efforts, I was failing to escape from the pattern followed by so many Western would-be do-gooders. Should I give money to the beggar at my gate, should I bargain at the market, should I buy bananas from this person on the corner, should I hire another housekeeper I don't actually need just to give someone a job? Every question I had seemed fraught, unanswerable; going outside the gate, or even the front door, meant facing these questions, embodied in real people: here is a man desperate to sell me something carved out of wood, here is another telling me that his wife gave birth to twins and then died, and can he have some money for formula; there is my Malawian neighbor calling out that this man is a liar, here are some children asking to come inside the gates and shake papayas from the tree in my yard. Increasingly, I drew the curtains against the light, against the need and the poverty and my own complicated connection to it all.

"It was like a *miscarriage*, okay?" I said, a little too loudly, and everyone at the table, all male, all clergy, some bearded and plaid clad and bespectacled in the hipster fashion, froze over their kale-and-lean protein salads and craft beers. A moment before, one of the pastors asked me about Malawi, and I told him that it hadn't gone well and had ended badly: with students bringing forth credible accusations of sexual abuse by several of the theological college faculty, with accusations of gross financial deception on the part of one faculty member, with rumors and evidence of many kinds of abuses all through the churches, and, in and through it all, with parasites and malaria and almost unbearable stress on our family.

"What good do you think came out of it?" the pastor asked.

I said I didn't know.

"Well, surely," he continued, "surely you must have done some good, planted some seeds; made some inroads for the gospel . . ."

That's when I cut him off.

Miscarriage.

At the other end of the table, one of the men, blue-eyed, bearded, drew his eyebrows together and up.

"There's a lot of pain in that word," he said.

"There is," I said. "Thank you."

When I went to settle up for my own salad and beer, the waitress told me that the blue-eyed bearded man, who had left early, had already paid: tip and all.

Sometimes the transformative power of a vessel fails to be realized. The wrong sorts of bacteria wind up in the milk, and instead of souring pleasantly and thickening into yogurt, it becomes a toxic sludge. When that happens, when milk is poured out instead of preserved, it is painful. When seeds lie dormant in dark soil, or among stones, you cannot see the promise of germination, and digging it up only makes chances worse. So you wait. You wait, and try to hope.

I made my enormous pot with Gloria and Fatima's help—a *msugo*, meant to hold water and keep it cool. *Like a refrigerator for the village*, Gloria joked, since villages aren't electrified and refrigerators are luxury items for the Malawian 1 percent. My *msugo* survived the fire without cracking, and I brought it back to my Malawian home in the city, filled it with soil, and planted it with young plants that, thanks to the heat and humidity, seemed to grow before my eyes: earthen vessels bearing earth, holding fragile life, making transformation and growth possible. Before we left the pottery lodge, Gloria used a length of bright African fabric to wrap my hair just as hers was wrapped. On our last night there, the choir from the village Anglican church—Gloria's church—came, and she pulled me into the mix of singing, dancing people, before we sat to eat.

"I will see you again?" Gloria asked.

"I hope so."

I left Malawi, and the pots were too heavy to take with me. I gave them, full of soil and blossoming with plants, to my Malawian neighbor. "I will enjoy them," she assured me. "I will enjoy them and remember you."

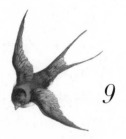

THE ODDS

*Science is the invaluable handmaiden of theology in
that it tells us how astonishing and gigantically elusive are all
the particulars of existence. And nothing is more unfathomable
than ourselves, individually and collectively, at any given
moment and from the earliest beginning of human time.*

MARILYNNE ROBINSON, *THE GIVENNESS OF THINGS*

Our house in Malawi had a playroom so well
stocked with LEGOs that once a little German
boy, the son of some missionaries, had to be dragged away
from it crying and screaming in his father's arms. Just seeing
the bounty of my children's toys set off in him a fit of envy
so terrific that it necessitated his being put directly to bed

upon returning to his own home. A certain gleam appears in many visitors' eyes when they take in the sheer number of LEGOs in our home: many secondhand, some in jumbled-up boxes, many tidily sorted into compartments, and scores built into models of castles and temples and vehicles of all kinds. Hundreds of LEGO minifigures stand at roll call on plastic building platforms.

When he was three and a half, my firstborn, Aidan, slipped on a wet supermarket floor in Paris as we shopped for a picnic we'd planned for later that evening. We lived in Scotland at the time, and Tim had a scholarship to study for a month in Paris. I froze when I heard that cry: it was like no other he'd ever made, and I *knew*. Within moments, the little leg was hot, red, and already misshapen; he was sweating hard. Only Tim could ride in the ambulance with him, so I stayed behind with my mother, who was visiting, and Graeme, who was a baby.

We waited in the apartment for news from the hospital: broken in two places, spiral fractures, plaster up to the thigh. *What do you do with a three-year-old boy who can't move?* I wondered. Aidan was rarely still in those days, unless he was asleep or being read to; he radiated energy and was constantly talking and moving. Even in toddlerhood, before he could walk unsupported, he insisted on walking the full mile to Tim's office, holding on to my hand, tiny step by tiny step.

Doing *something* while we waited for their return seemed better than staying in the apartment we were renting, and I had an idea: my mother and I would walk with Graeme to a little toy shop—I found it in my Fodor's *Paris* guide—and buy Aidan his first set of LEGOs. *That's a toy you can play with sitting still*, I reasoned. We purchased a bin of LEGOs and a bin of the larger, baby-safe version, DUPLOs, for Graeme, along with one minifigure for Aidan, since, as far as I was concerned, it was never much fun to construct buildings or vehicles if there were no people to use them, and Aidan felt similarly; his favorite toy to that point was a small digger that came with a small construction worker figure.

After the first painful, sleepless night, Aidan sat up in bed and built with LEGOs on a tray. Soon, the whole traumatic episode of the broken leg was transformed into the story of "how Aidan became a major LEGO enthusiast." A little more than a year later, Aidan's second broken leg coincided with his birthday, and we realized it would be awful to give him the bike we'd purchased. That birthday became remembered as "the birthday I broke my leg and got the LEGO fire truck." In this way we have measured moments and days, joyful and sad, in terms of LEGOs. Snapping bricks together, one at a time, piece by piece, my boys follow instructions occasionally but mostly create their own designs, replicating buildings and vehicles and scenes encountered in real life and in the pages of books: the LEGO airport security line with its metal detectors and queues of tired travelers appeared after we'd taken a series of trips, the LEGO Pequod with a peg-legged Ahab climbing the rigging after we'd read a children's adaptation of *Moby-Dick*. LEGOs, Tim likes to say, are more than a toy: they are an expressive medium, and with them my boys have exercised their creative minds and nimble fingers for thousands of hours, making hundreds of different creations; whole worlds, brick by brick.

I don't build much with LEGO, but I understand the appeal. My own hands are often busy with needles and yarn, and I like the endless possibilities of knitting: sticks and string and a few basic moves and I can make blankets and sweaters and socks and teddy bears. For as much as we spent time quietly reading or writing or thinking, we have, in our little family, the urge to make and do: to conceive of something and bring it forth into the world; to get our feet wet, travel far, make artifacts. Hence the endless LEGO models, the vegetable gardens and the compost, the ceramics and baking and outdoor sports. I don't think this is particularly unusual. I suspect many of us itch to do more with our finely engineered fingers and marvelous opposable thumbs than swipe at screens and tap on keyboards.

One of the best things about models and toys built from LEGOs is this: if and when you drop them, and they break, they can, with some diligence, be put back together again.

In between Aidan's first and second broken legs, his little brother, Graeme, also had a broken leg. All my life I've known that I had a genetic disorder known as osteogenesis imperfecta (OI), commonly known as brittle bone disease. I inherited it from my mom, who inherited it from her father, Harold, who inherited it from his mother, Jennie. My mother broke at least a dozen bones before the age of thirteen; my grandfather had broken many bones, and my great-grandmother, who died before my mother was born, had endured pain, disfigurement, and disability simply from having given birth to my grandfather and his younger brother. I didn't break many bones—partly because I was, as a child, uninterested in much physical activity beyond that which was necessary—and while I had more bruises, stress fractures, and sprains than other kids (and much less strength and agility), I didn't give OI much thought. When my obstetrician insisted that I see a genetic counselor as soon as possible, I shrugged off her concern. Everything, I was sure, would be fine.

Then came the year of the broken legs and several years of sprained ankles, and, of course, the many bruises, and, with all that, inappropriate jokes about child abuse and questions about whether or not our kids drank milk or took calcium. I was no longer sure that everything would be fine. Tim is tall and strong, and his nieces and nephews were sturdy little kids who could tumble in gymnastics and on their trampoline, kids whose parents and uncles could toss them playfully in the air. Ours were tiny, easily bruised, and slow to learn to walk, and all of that was because of me, because of the genes I gave them. I hated having to tell people to be careful when picking up our kids; it made me seem even more neurotically overprotective than I actually am. But kids with OI can't roughhouse like most kids.

One of the clinical markers of OI is blue sclera: what's usually called the "whites" of people's eyes appear blue due to the defect or deficit in the body's production of collagen—the protein that holds human bodies together and gives strength and structure to bone and muscle, skin and tendon. The whites of my eyes are blue because the "white"—the sclera—is made of collagen; without enough collagen the blue of the veins beneath glows through. Newborns sometimes have bluish sclera that change to white later as the sclera plump up with normal collagen, so when each of my babies was born, I scrutinized their eyes regularly, waiting for the day when their sclera would fade to pure white, like Tim's. First Aidan's stayed blue, then Graeme's, and my stomach rose under my ribs with that familiar nausea of fear and guilt.

"Well," my mom said. "Maybe it's getting milder each generation. Maybe it's just a trait now, like regular eye color." I wasn't convinced.

I've cringed a little when people exclaim how much my boys look like me—especially when people say that they have my eyes. Yes, they have my eyes, and I have my mother's, and she has her father's, and he had his mother's, and we all have the eyes of everyone who shares this rare genetic defect.

When I discovered that Ellen, a colleague and friend I'd only known online also, improbably, had OI, we exchanged pictures. *Yup*, she said, *we kind of look alike in that OI-ish way.* We became friends in real life, too, and have been for years now. And I love that she and I look something like family.

My mom and dad didn't plan on having children. It wasn't just the OI, but that was part of it. Both my grandfathers left their families in 1968, and both their families had discouraging patterns of mental illness and addiction. Practicing a little homespun eugenic theory over pizza in their favorite joint by Queens College, they decided to be childless.

But really, I always *wanted to be a mommy*, my mom says.

Best mistake I ever made! My dad jokes.

Yes: they'd decided to marry and to be childless, but they were also young and not inexperienced in the ways of the world, so despite belonging to a church that exhorted premarital chastity, my mom found herself to be in the family way a few weeks after she'd broken up with my dad.

My mother's doctors were adamant that she should have an abortion. Their understanding of the bone disorder wasn't great—the genetics and subtypes of the whole business weren't as well understood then as they are now, and my parents were assured that I would be born with bones already broken, if I wasn't in fact born dead. My mom, the doctor said, could expect to spend the rest of her life using a wheelchair after her spine collapsed or her pelvis broke or she was otherwise maimed by the birth, as her grandmother Jennie had been by the birth of my mother's uncle. My mother's family agreed. Get the abortion: safe, legal, merciful, therapeutic.

My father asked her not to.

My mother said it wasn't up to him, said she didn't have to talk to him.

My father said he knew that. He knew that what he was asking was in no way fair, and that the cost to her was incalculably greater than the cost to him, that if there were a way for him to carry the burden of a possibly broken child—he had seen pictures of people with severe forms of OI who must use wheelchairs all the time; who have tiny, crumpled bodies and suffer physical pain and the pain of the ignorance and prejudice of the able-bodied—and the burden of a possibly broken body himself, he would take it on, in his own flesh, which, of course, he could not. It was hers to bear, and hers alone. *I don't have any real right to ask this, but I am asking: please, please don't do this. If you are disabled by this, I will take care of you for the rest of my life. Please.*

Something shifted, fluttered open. She gave her consent. She really wasn't too worried, she said; she had a hunch everything was going to be all right. She ate meatball sandwiches with such regularity that the lady at the pizzeria said she was sure the baby would turn out to look like a meatball, and she grew very, very round. *I didn't really want the abortion*, she's told me. *That's what everybody else wanted for me. But I wanted you. I was so happy. I wanted a girl* so badly *and I got you.* Her orthopedist was furious, and, with scant consent, her obstetrician sterilized her the day I was born, when she was twenty-one years old. My dad paced and fretted and rushed in to count my fingers and toes as I lay alone in a box with big signs warning against anyone touching me lest I prove particularly breakable, which, all things considered, I'm not.

I am conscious, every day or nearly so, of how heavily the odds are stacked against any one person's existence, including my own. Never mind the yawning cosmos, think of the millions of sperm and hundreds of eggs and imponderable combinations thereof, of the thousands of minutes and glances and encounters, planned or chanced, of the dozens of ways things can go wrong in body and mind, of the choices and decisions whether rash and considered, of the fears and the labor and the pain overcome, of the courage and grit required to deliver a child, one child, *this* child, from the dark waters of the womb to the light and air of this world. I do not know how it is that we forget, that I forget, to look upon every human being I meet with something very near to reverence, if not reverence indeed. So many elements intersect to bring each one of us into being. That it happens imperfectly is less remarkable than the fact that it happens at all. The womb, the work and consent and strength of a woman, is the mother country from which we, all of us, have sojourned. We are wholly, equally holy.

There is privilege in this story. Not everyone has adequate health care and supportive partners. It doesn't always turn out all right. Sometimes it turns out so wrong. Women do die from childbirth injuries, and babies are born without ever taking a break, and the things we fear most do sometimes happen. Even within the subtype of OI that runs in our family, people suffer more and more severely broken bones. My friend Ellen has suffered more broken bones and surgeries than all my affected family members put together. It could be so much worse. I think about that constantly.

Still, I felt, and sometimes feel, a creeping sense of guilt when one of my kids gets a brutal-looking bruise from nothing in particular, or sore feet from a long-ish walk. I want to blame myself for giving them these genes. *No*, Tim says. *That's not how it works.* They are who they are, and I am who I am, and I am their mother, for better and worse. We are a family, and every family has got something.

On a winter's night not long ago, Tim, Aidan, Graeme, and I piled together with blankets on the couch, watching a documentary about LEGOs that only those already converted to the cult of LEGOs could love. I was busily knitting, making little woolen pants for a nephew not yet born. The documentary chronicled the history of the brick, the way LEGOs are used in group therapy settings, and what the LEGO design process looks like. My favorite part, however, was the spot with a mathematics professor who has calculated how many different ways there are to combine six LEGO bricks: nine million, one hundred thousand, seven hundred sixty-five. The possibilities inherent in a set of LEGOs, the professor suggested, are for all practical purposes, infinitely variable.

I cried when the two pink lines appeared on the stick in the bathroom at Target, and I cried throughout the pregnancy. Tim and I were planning to have children "someday," but certainly not *yet*. We thought we should wait until we each finished a few more graduate degrees and had wonderful, secure jobs in higher education. I was only twenty-three, and we'd been married for just a year and a half. Then—how many twists and turns in people's stories are now preceded by this phrase?—I started reading articles on the Internet about the birth control pill, which I was then taking every day, and I started feeling weird about it, like it wasn't as natural and maybe not as spiritual as, say, natural family planning. I hear that NFP works really well for some people, but I conceived my first son on a day when my chance of conceiving was, according to the data, less than 3 percent.

Still a sort of newlywed, I fretted over the change in our relationship that the baby would bring ("Will we still be best friends when the baby comes, Tim? Will we still be *best friends*?") I didn't like how only I got to be pregnant, and how we couldn't really share it. No one said "*we're* pregnant" in those days, and if they had I wouldn't have said it anyway because it isn't true: pregnancy is a condition almost as mysterious and inward as thought itself, and as such it is borne alone. Later, marveling over the very perfection of his existence—the *himness* of him—we delighted that God, hormones, and faulty family planning had given us *this specific person*, because if we'd waited for those great jobs in academia, we might still be waiting. And then, or at some other time, some other sperm might have joined with some other egg and we wouldn't ever have known who we were missing. But that line of reasoning gets tangled fast: we wouldn't have *Aidan*, and that's the point.

Of all the possible outcomes of the combination of my genes and Tim's, of my parents' genes and his, of our four sets of grandparents and eight sets of great-grandparents and back behind them, here we were, four people, huddled together in the glow of a screen, under the warmth of blankets, pondering the meaning of the infinite as applied to LEGO. Infinite. Going on forever, somehow, improbably, like the cosmos itself. Elements broken apart, put back together, assembled, reassembled, always. *Our existence, as individuals and as a family*, I thought, *is so unlikely that it's completely absurd.* The only response was to put down my knitting, nestle deeper into the blankets, and pull my boys closer.

Somewhere Aidan and Graeme heard or read that when a bone breaks and then heals, it's stronger in the spot where it was broken; thicker, the way scarred skin is thicker than the skin around it. Armed with that knowledge, they've declared themselves lucky, for, having been broken, they have grown stronger. I wish they could be stronger without having first to be broken. I wish their family tree did not lean so perilously over the seas of madness and melancholy into which so many of their forebears and mine have tumbled and struggled, with varying degrees of success, to paddle out from. Then, too, I wish they could grow mature and wise without facing adversity of any kind, but we all know how that goes. So I grudgingly reject the nonexistent "what could have been" and try to embrace what is—all the millions upon billions of variables that allowed their existence and their dad's and mine. When I consider it, I'm unspeakably grateful for this fragile shelter of togetherness, this family that we're constructing together, piece by piece, in this world of endless shifting and breaking and regrowth and change.

On their thirty-fifth wedding anniversary, my parents came to Tim and the boys' first LEGO fan convention exhibition. They'd built a Viking island populated by dragons, based on a popular story and film, in which seemingly ferocious dragons are tamed by kindness. My contribution was a blue satin cloth for the display table that provided the illusion of a LEGO sea. I sat knitting behind the table, fielding design questions from endless faces in the crowd as my mother and father and husband and sons strolled in various combinations in the convention center, among the tens of thousands of people and hundreds of thousands of LEGO bricks and figures. My anxious mind flitted about, wondering where we'd hide if a mass shooter entered the building, what would happen if one of the boys got separated from my parents in the crowd, and what kind of microbes might be swarming the convention center. We all gathered around a table for lunch, a moment of calm in the LEGO storm. My mom built a small set with Graeme. My dad and Aidan assembled minifigures depicted with historically accurate clothing and equipped with historically accurate accessories. Later, my mom said, she'd realized that it had been the perfect way to celebrate their anniversary.

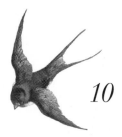

BAPTIZE

It is a characteristic of God to overcome evil with good.

Jesus Christ therefore, who himself overcame evil with good, is our true Mother. We received our 'Being' from Him and this is where His Maternity starts—And with it comes the gentle Protection and Guard of Love which will never cease to surround us.

Just as God is our Father, so God is also our Mother.

JULIAN OF NORWICH, *REVELATIONS OF DIVINE LOVE*

Why does the Bible, and why do some Christians, speak of a second birth—of being "born again"?

For some, the phrase carries a whiff of misogyny. In *Sexism and God Talk*, the feminist Catholic theologian Rosemary Radford Ruether suggests that male theologians, insisting on the necessity of a second birth, imply that the first birth is contaminating—the life given by the woman is reconceived by men as the source of death. Fear and hatred of female bodies, she argues, is behind the Roman Catholic emphasis on baptism at the hands of a male priest (which is why midwives, who baptized babies who died just after birth, were held in grave suspicion in the Middle Ages) as well the evangelical emphasis on being "born again."

The eighteenth-century French priest and theologian Nicolas Malebranche wrote presciently of the intimate connection between expectant mother and unborn child—postulating something very near to what contemporary science has indicated to be the case: that even the mother's state of mind can and does influence the baby's. He finds a theological lesson in this naturalistic observation: *because of this communication [between mother and child] it must also be that* sin comes from woman, *that through her we are subject to death, and that our mother has conceived us in iniquity.* In context,

Malebranche is taking St. Paul one step further; where Paul writes that sin entered the world "through one man," Malebranche wants to be sure women share in the blame. His emphasis on the contaminating effects of the mother's body and mind on the baby she houses may well reflect the fear and loathing of bodies in general—and female bodies in particular—that has long dogged Christianity and Western thought more generally. "Reason," claims the philosopher Sara Ruddick, means "mind-over-body," and to be "reasonable" is to put "mind over matter." In Western philosophy, she argues, mind and reason are coded as masculine, while bodies—particularly female bodies, with their troubling tendency to bleed, leak milk, and exhibit insufficient individuation by hosting other tiny human bodies—stand for all that reason is not.

All this is certainly more gnostic than authentically Christian, since the Jewish and Christian Scriptures are clear that God made the world, this world, and that God loves it all and calls it good. Nonetheless, the denial of the body has a long history in Christendom. Catholic teaching officially has it that Jesus somehow escaped Mary's body without passing through her vagina. The second-century apocryphal Gospel known as the *Protoevangelium of James* imagines Jesus' birth happening this way: "A great light appeared in the cave so that our eyes could not endure it. And by little and little that light withdrew itself until the young child appeared: and it went and took the breast of its mother Mary."

There is no anguish, no blood, no vagina in this birth story; the baby Jesus simply manifests after an overwhelming light recedes: here's the likely source of the image, from the Catholic tradition, of Jesus simply appearing, miraculously and painlessly, outside Mary's womb "without opening the passage." Clearly, it was written by a man.

Addressing Mary herself, St. Augustine wrote, "In conceiving thou wast all pure, in giving birth thou wast *without pain*." He should have consulted his mother, Monica, on the matter. She might have had a different idea. That the birth of Jesus was painless and vagina-free was confirmed at the Council of Trent, in which Catechism it is written: "To Eve it was said: In sorrow shalt thou bring forth children. Mary was exempt from this law, for preserving her virginal integrity inviolate she brought forth Jesus the Son of God without experiencing, as we have already said, any sense of pain."

Yet the scandal of the incarnation is that God became a human not by being beamed down from on high but by being born in the usual way: clinging, as a bundle of cells, to the blood-rich inner wall of Mary's womb, floating in the amniotic bubble inside Mary's uterus, that astonishingly strong and expansible muscle making room within her body, her hospitable body, for God the Son to develop limbs, heart, brain, fingernails, earlobes, eyelashes. The scandal of the incarnation is that a woman—we might even be tempted to refer to Mary as a girl, she was so young—was in labor with God. *A girl was in labor with God.* She groaned and sweated and arched her back, crying out for her deliverance and finally delivering God, God's head pressing on her cervix, emerging from her vagina, perhaps tearing her flesh a little; God the Son, her Son, covered in vernix and blood, the infant God's first breath the close air of crowded quarters, the iron and animal and tart and fecal smell of a birthing suite; God the Son, her Son, pressed to her bare breast, baby lips parted, tongue searching and seeking, the two of them still connected by the umbilicus, God's placenta detaching, no longer needed, as Mary's womb involuted, the two of them separating, then connecting again as God the Son, her Son, drank deeply from his mother. *Drink, my beloved. This is my body, broken for you.*

I do not, of course, presume to know how it was, but if the incarnation is real, then it began as all human life begins, emerging, as Augustine so indelicately put it, from "between feces and urine." It began with Mary's bloated and tender breasts, with her swelling body and an aching back, with her exhaustion and hunger and thirst. It began when her contractions stopped being exciting—an intimation that the moment of birth was closer now than when she first consented—and began to be grueling, when she cried out *my God, my God, have you forsaken me?*

But it began, truly, when she consented and not before, for Mary is no passive vessel. No mere container for the divine, she is an active co-creator with God.

As a Protestant, I grew up knowing that I was not supposed to venerate Mary, because that's what the Catholics did; secretly, I wanted to as well, not because I thought I needed an intercessor between Jesus and myself, but because she was a girl, a woman, like me. I do not pray to Mary, but I accord her honor in my prayer. When, in the liturgy, we confess our salvation by Jesus' wounds and our healing by Jesus' blood, I acknowledge her body and blood, too. I look at her image for comfort and in adoration, for not to wonder at Mary is, I believe, not to wonder at the incarnation itself.

Premodern conceptions of reproduction—difficult as it is to believe—didn't always imagine women's bodies as having an integral role. Instead, in ancient Near Eastern accounts, the man's seed is deposited into the woman's soil; she does not contribute to the formation of the seed, to its essence—it was thought to contain all that it needed to become what it is to become—but merely furnishes a place for it to grow. For millennia, people believed that each baby grew from a homunculus—a microscopic but complete human being, deposited by the father in the mother's womb. Lacking the insight that women do, in fact, contribute more than just a toasty hideout for a fully formed but infinitesimal human, people have been inclined, and sometimes *are* inclined, to regard women as passive fetus containers, as incubators.

I have heard the Annunciation—when Gabriel tells Mary of the immanent incarnation, that she has been chosen by God to bear God—described as a form of divine rape, akin to the sorts of obscenities perpetrated upon human women by masculine members of the Greek and Roman pantheons. But reading the Annunciation as if it were Zeus's rape of Leda fails to take into account the story's most indispensable and obvious details: namely, that Mary delights in the role she is offered and accepts it. She gives her consent—*let it be with me according to your word.* Let it be.

"Obedience is not a virtue unless there exists the genuine possibility of not obeying. The Mary of the Gospels is, above all, a paradigm of the choice of all women, writes Tikva Frymer-Kensky. "Pregnancy always involves choice, and the choice is not always easy." (Frymer-Kensky assumes that women always have the choice of abortion.) Mary consents to stretch marks and sagging breasts. Mary consents to endure the discomfort of pregnancy and the agony of birth. Mary consents to shoulder the risk of hemorrhaging with no hope of a transfusion, of succumbing to puerperal sepsis in a world that knows nothing of germs, much less of antibiotics. For the joy set before her, anchored in hope, in God's promise to deliver, Mary consents. She risks. She wades through the waters. God troubles them. She comes through the other side.

Twice now I have stayed on the campus of a Catholic abbey and university in Minnesota, a place where, it seems, water and land are indistinctly separate; where there is land there is also lake, and one seems to extend into another. It's beautiful: sunlight blinking on the riffles of the water, fish darting among lily leaves, baby turkey vultures, not yet homely, nodding along the banks. A trail runs for a mile or so along one of these lakes to a small chapel—the Stella Maris chapel. *Stella Maris* is Latin for "Star of the Sea," and has traditionally stood as an invocation of Mary, the mother of Jesus, as a protecting and guiding figure for seafarers, likely because mariners employ stars straightforwardly as navigational tools.

Maritime metaphors have long been beloved of Christians, who have imagined the journey of life as something like a sea voyage; for those who seek refuge there, church serves as an ark or a lifeboat; faith is perhaps a scrap of floating wreckage to cling to; grace, the mysterious lightness that grants buoyancy; hope, the anchor that keeps the seafarer moored even through turbulence. I don't know what love's maritime metaphor might be, but I suspect it is to be found in presence:

the presence of fellow travelers, or even the dream or memory of such presence, or the sense, however fleeting, of the presence of God. The central part of many traditionally designed Western churches—where most of the congregation sits—is known as the *nave*, from the Latin, *navis*: ship.

When I first visited the Stella Maris chapel, I didn't notice much in the architecture that made me think of a boat. I was disappointed. I noticed the stained-glass windows, the cobalt blue of my favorite variety of beach glass, but unclouded and rippled and populated sparsely with images suggesting a child's idea of fish. I liked how the lead framework of each window is open to the outside so that in the chapel one is not sequestered from the outside, the surrounding lake and trees and air not cut off from this sacred space. Only when I returned a couple of years later did I notice that the ceiling beams strongly suggest the hull of a wooden ship. And near the starboard bow there stands a sculpture of Mary—of pregnant Mary.

For several days before I trekked out to the chapel I'd sculpted Mary's figure in my mind. I imagined a full-figured Mary, a forty-one weeks pregnant Mary, Mary with swollen breasts and swollen ankles, Mary so pregnant she can't breathe with her mouth closed, Mary who just wants to put her feet up, Mary who has reached the point at which enduring labor becomes preferable to the prospect of remaining pregnant. But the Mary in the chapel is a slender, girlish Mary, a lithe and willowy Mary who might be featured on the cover of a prenatal fitness magazine. I realized that what I'd wanted to see was something like the lavish womanly figures one sees in ancient fertility idols; figures that are embarrassingly frank about fruitfulness, or potential fruitfulness: all curves and no angles. Mary *was* probably a teenager. Maybe she was scrawny.

I was still a scrawny teenager when I began to detest all curves, beginning, perhaps, with those in my spine. My scoliosis was severe by the time it was noticed. I was fourteen, fifteen, sixteen, and the curve in my spine was just one of many emerging curves that I regarded as in need of regulation. I equated womanly bodies with bodies that were no longer ideal, as I believe many people unconsciously do, and this was confirmed by middle-aged ladies whose compliments on my slenderness were accompanied by nostalgia for their own teenage bodies and prophecies that I wouldn't look like that forever, particularly not after I had children. Everywhere in popular culture and discourse, it seemed, the shape of womanliness, the shape of a mother, was a thing to dread; the pre- or early adolescent shape a thing for which to pine.

When I became pregnant at twenty-three, I was still afraid of being a woman, still worried about taking up space, still anxious about womanly curves. I felt myself rocking on turbulent seas in a flimsy dinghy, too afraid to call out to Jesus, asleep in the stern, unable to call out to the Star of the Sea, to find my way. I was a pregnant and frightened child, afraid to expand hospitably for the sake of my child. When I first saw the skinny pregnant Mary statue, I didn't like it. She didn't suggest that it is good to take up space, to be great with child, to be heavy: *gravid*, the medical Latin for pregnant, is the Latin word for *heavy*.

Then I looked back at my photo albums. I was a skinny pregnant person. My grandmother was a skinny pregnant person. *That statue looks like* you *did*, my friend pointed out, and it was true. But it is not only the strong and fertile-looking that can take up space, hold their own, and navigate rough waters. In the upside down logic of the Gospels, and of the Scriptures as a whole, *of course* it is a frail, too-young, too-small Mary who consents boldly, who chooses to stretch and bend and nearly to break her body to make room on this earth for God. When Julian of Norwich, the English mystic, saw a vision of Mary, she saw not a physically imposing woman but "a meek and simple maid, young, little more than a child, of the same bodily form as when she conceived." She looked, to Mother Julian, like the Stella Maris sculpture.

After Malawi, when I had been back in the United States for a year, an old friend, Eva, put out a call on social media to ask if anyone knew a doula in the area. I said I lived in the area and was a doula, and so I became hers. Over coffee, she told me that she preferred to have agency—"pain or discomfort seems so much worse if I don't have some kind of control," she said. "I want to give birth without any numbing, if possible, so that I'm not a body in a bed having things done *to* me." I understood. We talked about those passages in Isaiah where God is pictured as a mother actively struggling her baby into the world, and the detail in the crucifixion story that Jesus refused the sip of wine that might have numbed his agony, even as he had cried out for God to take his suffering away. There was dignity and courage in going through deep waters.

A few weeks later, Eva rocked and moaned and danced her way through the swells, floated and even napped through the moments of calm. She kept her body free from tension and fear; a textbook example of a woman well-practiced in the best technique of natural childbirth—and still it hurt. Her husband and I held her up. We wiped away the sweat and put the straw in her mouth so she could sip. We pressed on her back and let her pull our hands; she braced against us, rested against us. She gasped, *pray*, and we did. And then she was transfigured when her baby finally came and she lay back, holding him to her chest, still bleeding, cooing and laughter so quickly replacing tears and groaning. Her face, still damp and red with effort, glowed, absorbed in her baby's face, searching out its details. I stepped back quietly. It was almost too beautiful to look at, like transfiguration. *This is the miracle that saves the world*, I thought.

Once, I received Communion in a church where the celebrant employed a variety of complicated circumlocutions to avoid saying the word *blood*. I have heard and read that Christians ought to let go of that embarrassing notion that Christ's violent, bloody, painful death is what somehow secures salvation. To hold on to this idea, I've heard it said, perpetuates a culture tolerant of violence.

But Christ's death only appeared to be passive suffering and defeat. Jesus went to the cross "for the joy set before him." Jesus is strong in his weakness. He refused the wine. He healed a severed ear and spoke words of comfort and pardon even as his own broken body sweat blood, even as he cried out, naked and flayed before gawkers and mourners. He gushed blood and water as he died; the gush that, in a pregnant woman, announces imminent birth. "[He] was in labor for the full time until he suffered the sharpest pangs and the most grievous suffering that ever were or shall be," Julian of Norwich wrote of Christ as Mother, "and at last he died." Then he appeared, alive, to the women who clung to him as their teacher, as their friend, transformed enough that it took them a moment to recognize him, yet still bearing scars, the way my mom and many of my friends have scars on their bellies from cesarean sections. *If you cannot name blood in* CHURCH, I scrawled in my bulletin, *where CAN you name it?*

"Wholeness," writes Sara Ruddick, "means accepting the interlacing of promise and suffering, suffering and comfort, breaking apart and creation—and of each new life with some particular woman's painful labor."

The worst kind of pain is that which burns without the hope of cooling comfort, of ending, of relief. Such pain is a flood without the grace of an ark, or, at least, a high place, a rock upon which to rest, suffering and death without resurrection, labor without birth.

Hope: believing that some alleviation, some hand to hold or some hands to hold us, some ark, some higher place is always on its way, that our suffering, our struggle, our death, even, somehow generates life of some kind; leads to some homegoing, some rescue, some return: salvation. There's a bit of false etymology that's grown up around the word *hope*, and I like it, even though it's not true. *Hope*, some people have claimed, comes from the word for hoop. I like it because hope should be round. Hope, like wholeness, like holiness, yearns for healing, resolution, closure. Hope believes that the circle will indeed be unbroken, by and by.

PREVENT

Rachel cried there for her children not yet born
not yet soft-faced infants whose mothers melt to them.
In the field she stood to the wind,
transparent as her shadow,
and her flesh was with the soil.
Joseph and Benjamin already clods
and she cried for her children against the hills.
Rachel cried for her children
before they know how to cry
before they burst from the dust
to return to it.

RIVKA MIRIAM, *RACHEL CRIED THERE*

I insisted that we tell no one of the incident with the baby and the HIV-positive blood at the hospital until I'd gotten the all-clear, which I was all but certain was coming six or twelve weeks hence, thinking, primarily, that I did not want to worry my parents. Somehow, though, I let slip in another phone conversation with my mom that I'd caught a baby.

"You caught a baby!"

She was all disbelief and wonder.

"Well, sort of; it was out already, I just picked it up and put it on its mother," I said, trying to make it sound boring so she'd change the subject.

"Rachel! *Your hands were the first hands to touch that baby!*"

Her reverence suggested something sacramental—baptism, perhaps. Which, as I thought back to that baby in her little puddle of water and blood, her strong substance in my hands as I placed her slippery body on her mother's chest, didn't seem so off the mark.

"Isn't that what you *dreamed* of?"

It was true. For more than two years I'd trolled the websites of nurse-midwifery programs. "You'd be a natural," a family friend—herself a nurse—had said, watching me at the bedside of her dying mother, who'd been like a grandmother to me. I loved being with her in the quiet room, rubbing lotion into her papery hands, painting her nails, singing hymns and making one-sided conversation, remembering, I suppose, all those movies and books where the doctors and nurses tell family members to speak to the comatose since they can hear. But I didn't and don't have the stomach for the risk and responsibility of nursing. Still, each time I watched Malawian midwives palpate a pregnant belly and listen for the heartbeat, each time I saw their hands poised to catch a baby, emerging white-and-blue from the mother's body, arms and legs and mouth springing open to the world, I thought *I would do anything to get to be near this miracle.* But when it came down to it, I preferred to observe. I had no intention of bloodying my hands.

The large white antiretroviral pills came in a large white bottle, which I hid carefully in my desk drawer. Like virtually all *azungus* in Malawi, I had hired help, who would, I knew, recognize the large white bottle and fear what it represented. Erasing the stigma of HIV, and of the medicines that control it, has been a daunting task in places like Malawi, where influential pastors stand in the pulpit on World AIDS Day and tell people that if they have faith enough, they don't need to get tested or to take medicine. Tim and I heard this kind of thing with our own ears, from our own colleagues. I didn't want anyone whispering about what pills I might be taking, and why.

"How am I going to survive until I get the definitive results back?" I whispered to Tim as we lay in bed.

"I'm sure you're going to be fine."

"I wish someone could put me in a coma and wake me up when it turns out I am fine," I said.

Some European and American families living in Malawi didn't bother with malaria prevention and water filtration for themselves and their kids. They were fine with their kids going on school field trips to the government hospital where who knows what kind of microbes were swirling around. But we'd gotten all the extra vaccines, and we took malaria pills. We paid careful, disinfecting attention to little things, like shaving cuts, after a friend who'd lived for years in the jungles of Papua New Guinea warned us to do so. Even so, we drove around in cars—probably the most dangerous part of any trip in Africa, and also impossible to avoid. Almost from the first day, I wondered whether, in the calculation of risk versus benefit, there was any good reason for us to be there.

I lay in bed that Good Friday after popping my first anti-retroviral pills, damp and sticky and praying for the electricity to go back on and get our little fan going. I felt I was in exile, far from the familiar and the beloved in every imaginable way. Easter Sunday, and resurrection, seemed impossibly far away, if not, in fact, impossible.

The work we had officially come to Malawi to pursue—
teaching in a Presbyterian theological college—seemed
thwarted and difficult at every turn. Our roles were unclear,
conceived and outlined in a boardroom in Louisville, thousands of miles, both literally and conceptually, from our Malawian colleagues. Tim taught Bible and theology, and I taught
English composition and research methods, but even in our
classrooms we felt fairly useless. Our accents were hard for
our students to understand. Nothing we had to teach seemed
useful to them. "Mrs. Stone, please just give us a list of things
to do, one, two, three, to write a good term paper. Don't tell
us there are different points of view. Give us the *correct* point
of view!"

Everything I'd learned about postcolonialism in graduate
school came back to mind, though this, too, provided anything but easy answers. Great Britain had released Malawi as
an independent member of the Commonwealth more than
fifty years before we got there, but English was used everywhere officially and, in theory at least, in government schools,
to everyone's disadvantage: it is no one's first language and
also the language that everyone must master to get by, and
certainly to get ahead. England no longer ruled, but English
did, and so did outmoded British models of education, of

nursing, of policing, and just about everything else: people conforming themselves—and pressuring others to conform—to a language and to models utterly foreign and largely irrelevant. If I was not exactly perpetuating the continued colonization of the mind, I also wasn't doing much to help anyone resist it: my job was to help my students improve their English, and none of them had objections. Speaking English well could well be lucrative. Thinking about why this was so could well be risky.

It was easier to talk to the furniture makers, the potters, the painters, the farmers—the poorer people, those whose education had been nominal, or nonexistent, who possessed what a Zen master might call "beginner's minds," minds open to possibility. Our seventy-two-year-old housekeeper, James, was skeptical that compost and chicken manure in place of chemical fertilizer would make our garden grow, but he tried it. A young man, Nasan, who painted and made screens and built a climbing structure for our boys to play on, eagerly learned basic carpentry from Tim. He was barely nineteen, and his young wife was expecting their first child. We'd lean on the fence and talk about children. His excitement was effervescent. He built a little elevated playhouse, complete with a tiny thatched roof, and linked it to another small structure with a wooden and rope bridge. Passersby stopped to watch the playground taking shape in our yard and asked if Nasan would come and build something similar for them. I would sing Nasan's praises to whomever would listen. I was delighted, because reputation is everything in a place like Malawi, and Nasan was gifted and dutiful, fair and reliable. I could see his career taking shape in my mind. We loaned him money for a bicycle so he could stop spending money on the minibus from the village and take on more jobs.

The baby was born, and, to Nasan's delight, it was a boy. Nasan kept working for us to pay off the bicycle—he was so proud of that bicycle and the independence it represented, and Tim and the boys drove out to the village to meet his wife and the baby and to bring a gift: one hundred pounds of maize, as good or better than cash. He wanted Tim to name the baby—in effect, to be its godfather. It was an honor he gently declined; to name a baby is to take responsibility for its life and spiritual well-being, and how could he promise such a thing when we knew we wouldn't be in Malawi for long?

As it turned out, we would have been there long enough.

One morning, Tim's phone rang at 3 and it was Nasan. They had been visiting family near Mt. Mulanje, and the baby, just three months old, had been taken to the hospital, sick, and died as soon as they got there. He had to sell the bicycle to pay for the little funeral and the bus fare home.

"What did he die of?" I whispered.

"What do any of these babies die of?" Tim shrugged.

Poverty, of course, and the indifference of the wealthy.

We called Nasan and asked him to come around again, but his number changed, or his phone was lost, or he was ashamed of his debt, and after a while, people stopped asking who had built the beautiful play houses and climbing structure, and whether he could build another one for their children.

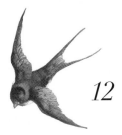

12

DIVE

It's a happy life, but someone is missing.

It's a happy life, and someone is missing.

ELIZABETH MCCRACKEN, *AN EXACT REPLICA*
OF A FIGMENT OF MY IMAGINATION

'm sad today," I told my Malawian neighbor Belinda.
"My friend from America had a baby, and the baby died."

"Unusual for you Americans. Normal for us. What happened?" She asked this without a trace of irony or bitterness as I explained that the baby had been born with certain organs underdeveloped, and that not even the best of Western medicine had been able to save him.

Having to face the death of children is, speaking historically and globally, the norm. When I think of that, I seem ridiculous to myself, with my litanies of fears about the health and safety of my children, or else I feel certain that I would have, in a more precarious age or place, been culled from the herd of humanity, swept away by debilitating grief. I read once about a woman who was committed to Dunning, a notorious Chicago asylum, over a century ago, after her baby died. The woman's great-grandson told the reporter that his great-grandmother had refused to let go of the dead baby, rocking it in her arms for days before she was hauled off to the asylum, where she too died. Infant mortality rates at the time suggest that this woman's loss was anything but unusual. Perhaps some women navigated the tempest of grief more successfully than others. Like most mothers, I have lived in fear of having to face this. I have felt sure I would not survive.

My grandmother barely survived the death of her baby Elise, but if Elise hadn't died, my mother probably wouldn't have been born, just a year and a half after the older sister she knew only from a pencil drawing died suddenly in the night. The apartment was being painted, and my grandmother didn't want the baby to breathe in the paint fumes, so she'd taken her to her paternal grandmother's house—to Jennie's house—for the night, and Elise hadn't woken up. Jennie, though disfigured from OI and arthritic, was skilled at tending babies; a business card of hers describes her as a "baby nurse." There was no discernable reason, no one to blame, though my grandmother had smoked through her pregnancy to avoid gaining weight (this was not discouraged) and had endured the surgical removal of an ovarian cyst while pregnant.

My grandmother was truly beautiful. Her large, green eyes were fringed with dark lashes and shadowed by straight brows. Her neck was long, but not overly long, and her face was heart shaped, high cheeked, and perfect: adorable in her youth and stunning in maturity. She never grew taller than 4'10" and had a petite and lovely figure. She sang, played the piano, spoke French—all beautifully—and submitted sheafs of poems to the *New Yorker*. I have found them, filed, with rejection notes clipped neatly to them.

Toward her later years, my grandmother resembled no one so much as the witch in Walt Disney's *Snow White*. Her hair was sparse, stringy, unwashed; teeth were missing. Her eyes, by then mostly lashless, bulged; the rest of her was sunken and yellowed, toenails and fingernails thickened and untrimmed. She smelled of solvents, of something you might use to strip old furniture of its finish. I cannot tell you of her beauty without telling you this. I cannot tell you this without telling you of her beauty.

She lived for so many years with a patient determination to end her life. She was "too chicken" to put a pistol to her head, she said. So she let vodka and cigarettes do it very slowly. The only thing that she feared in the afterlife, she said, was that she might be able to feel the worms eating her.

I have feared resembling my grandmothers and my great-grandmothers: the physical limitations, the mental instabilities, the addictions, the phobias. For years I have watched movies and plays with scenes of women going mad, and I have shivered in recognition, fearing that the time would come when I, too, would lose touch with reality, stolidly reject all outside help, and end it all quickly, with a bang, or quietly, with cigarettes and extra-extra-dry martinis, like my grandmother. For years I flinched when the phone rang at odd hours, terrified that it would be someone calling to tell me that my grandmother had died, or my grandmother herself, drunkenly crying or raving into the telephone.

Twice a year, my grandmother sat patiently and allowed my mother to try and convert her to Christianity. A thoroughly secular Jew, my grandmother hated that my mother had found religion, and found *that* religion, but my grandmother was tolerant and good-hearted and she knew it was an im-perative of my mother's evangelical faith that my mother at-tempt to convert her. "If there is a God," she said on one such occasion, "then I have a bone to pick with him."

My grandmother said that Elise was the most beautiful baby she had ever seen, and my grandmother was not one to hand out unmerited praise or to gush over babies. "Don't you want to see her again?" my mother would plead with her mother when I was still a child, believing that if she died unconverted, she wouldn't go to heaven and would never see Elise. But what kind of God would take the most beautiful baby as she slept in her crib? A weak and powerless God, or a sadistic and bloodthirsty God. God would not have left my grandmother without even a photograph of Elise. There is only a penciled sketch by Jennie, who wrote in the lower right corner: "Elise, as I remember her (from memory)."

"Did Grandma go for counseling?" I asked my mother, years after my grandmother was gone. "Yeah, 80-proof counseling," my mother snorted. After my grandmother drank herself so low that we had to call an ambulance, and then an extreme cleaning service, she came to live with us. I was fourteen. She had been through the worst part of detox and didn't drink at all. "I've joined the Prozac nation, dahling!" she announced. "I am *disgustingly* cheerful. I find myself saying 'good morning' to everyone." For a while, the only pints she polished off were Häagen-Dazs. But she moved back to her own apartment, and soon—when winter came? When her prescription ran out and she refused to fill it? When her demons came creeping back?—she sought the numbness of the bottle, and the corner liquor store resumed delivery of her standard order, brown-bagged, to her apartment door. She slipped money under the door. It added up to a gallon every five days. You could hear the ice tinkle in her glass through the phone.

I hadn't liked having her live with us, and I complained about her, and even now I fantasize that if I'd been more hospitable, I could have saved her. I had always wanted to save her. I would throw my arms around her in a fit of evangelistic fervor and beg her to "let Jesus into her heart." She would smile vaguely and pat my hair. She was a very good sport. Once, on a hot and humid September day, she carried a glass aquarium ten city blocks in her high heels because it was my turn to have the class hamster for the weekend. She played endless rounds of Go Fish and Candy Land, and later of Boggle and Scrabble. When I finished my first *New York Times* crossword puzzle, I called her right away. (She could do the Sunday puzzles with her fountain pen.) "Oh, congratulations, dahling!" By then she had become mostly a voice on the phone; she didn't want us to see how she was letting herself decay once again. But we talked. When I was captivated by the musical *Sweeney Todd*, we talked it over: the criminal madness, the injustice, the impossibility of untangling who is ultimately culpable, morally speaking. "Grandma! I can't believe the ending!" I exclaimed.

"Oh, dahling. I love your youth. I love hearing your surprise," she said.

It is strange, or it is not at all strange, that I associate with that grotesque tale of selfishness and deception and true love lost and lives ruined and preposterously twisted by factors outside anyone's control. When I think of *Sweeney Todd* I think of my grandmother, the two of us clutching our phones with but a few miles of city between us, wishing the story could have turned out differently.

When I was eleven and living way out on Long Island, by the water, my mother cried after my grandmother boarded the bus and returned to her apartment in the city.

"Are you crying about her toenails?" I asked.

My grandmother's toenails, which during that visit I had opportunity to scrutinize, had been thick, yellowed, and so long that they were curling. It was difficult to see how she had been able to walk or to wear a shoe. To be trimmed at all, they had first had to be soaked. The strange part was that my grandmother at that point had not yet given herself over to ruin. She still dressed nicely, colored her hair, accessorized her outfits.

"It's the toenails and it's . . ." my mother paused and hunted for the words "because she doesn't . . . take care of herself."

In those days the church where my father was pastor had in its membership covenant a clause about abstaining from alcohol. Later, this prohibition fell away, and when it did, it was generally discovered that no one had ever been especially adherent to it anyway. But my mother is a very truthful soul, even to the point of only hesitantly allowing me to use her Costco card without her there alongside, and she felt then that to have her alcoholic mother imbibing under the roof of the Baptist parsonage would have been a sinful deception.

She told my grandmother that she couldn't drink at our house anymore, which meant that my grandmother didn't come to that house again. And she told me, finally: "Grandma's an alcoholic."

It was a cold slap. I was indignant, affronted, pained, because I somehow thought that God, or Christianity, required me to hold her, or my affections for her, at arm's length because of her "sins." I wept because I wanted to go on loving her, and I thought God did not approve. I thought God wanted me to withhold my love and acceptance until she mended her ways. It didn't occur to me for the longest time that not loving people because they weren't perfect was pretty nearly the opposite to any Christian understanding of God that holds any water.

"I should have poured the drinks for my mother," my mother said, years after her mother had died. "Not because I condoned the alcoholism, but because she *was going* to drink—and it would have been better for her not to be alone." Sometimes, in my dreams, I play Scrabble with my grandmother, and we drink cocktails.

I was twenty-two when I said my last goodbye to my grandmother. She was buoyed immensely by the knowledge that she was so close to death; death was what she'd been angling for all these long years. It wasn't that she thought she was headed to "a better place," or that she thought she was about to "see Elise in heaven." Her spirits were lifted by the knowledge that the heavy task of living would soon be over. I can understand how she felt that way. I sometimes wondered that my faith was exactly what she believed it to be: a crutch, and not always a very sturdy one at that.

Could not, for example, the idea of resurrection simply been invented because the finality of death—the death of a Messiah, the death of a six-month-old baby, one's own death—is too much to take? The church culture of my childhood insisted that there should be something very different about Christians, such that unconverted people would notice that special something and wonder what it was. But I was so much like my grandmother. I had a few bones to pick with God, too. It was only years later, as I listened to an interview with the Holocaust survivor Elie Wiesel while pinning diapers on the clothesline, that I realized that picking bones with God has a long and venerable tradition. Job did it. The psalmists did it, and Jesus too. There are no answers to our questions, only the assurance of God's presence everywhere, in the weirdest and wildest places—on a mountain when the wild goats give birth, in the depths of the sea when the whales sing. There is only—and in Christianity, this is everything—the astonishing humility of God in taking on flesh. Of making a woman's body his home, of being squeezed and pushed and grunted into the world, of suffering hunger and loneliness, humiliation and death. Of sharing our lot. God's presence, Christ's compassion, so often shown to us when one person reaches toward another in empathy, in companionship, in love.

My grandmother, as I have said, played games with me. I try to do this with my children, though games sometimes fill me with existential dread. Why are we subjecting ourselves to these arbitrary constraints? Does it really matter who builds the longest road or places a Z on a triple-letter score? And it's all kind of a waste of time. It's a short walk from these thoughts to thoughts about life itself. Why bother getting out of my pajamas if I'm just going to get into them again? Why make the bed when I have to unmake it? Why keep on living when life is guaranteed to be hard and sad and to end in death?

On better days—indeed, on most days, thanks be to God and to my antidepressants—I can see that, in fact, to regard life as a game isn't to see it as futile or arbitrary at all. The world is not a series of solemn necessities, as both religion and science in different ways would occasionally have it, unfolding determinedly at the behest either of natural selection or of a sovereign, joyless God. To the contrary, the only explanation I find at all satisfying is that it—all of it—exists purely for the Creator's joy and delight, and for ours. It's an astonishing gift to have the capacity to enjoy things that we don't, strictly speaking, need, and games reveal that more clearly than just about anything. So what if we can't play the game forever, and there is no guarantee of winning, and there is always, always chance?

I know my grandmother sometimes felt bored and distracted when she played with me, just as I do sometimes when I play with my children. She played anyway. And memory of that—her willingness to play the game—fills me with love for her, and for my children, these people who carry a bit of her within themselves, as I do. The memory of that makes me want to play the game, and play it well. My grandmother hadn't really wanted children, and hadn't really known what do with the children she had. "What business did she have even *having* children," I asked my mom once. "I don't know," she said. "But I'm glad I'm here."

There were very few things to salvage from her apartment at the end, but her beautiful teak mid-century piano, cleaned and tuned, sits in my dining room, and when my son plays it, his eyes sparkle. He loves music and games and jokes and food; he loves *life*. Sometimes I sip liqueur from one of the tiny crystal glasses that were hers, and we use her wedding silver on holidays or when I need more place settings. For a long time, if I put my nose very close to the piano keys, I could smell my grandmother's cigarettes. When the smell faded, I bought a pack of her brand and put it next to an ashtray on top of the piano, under her portrait. "You know, I smoked a few cigarettes with her before she died," my mother reminded me. Sometimes, on the anniversary of her death, we light up together, glad we're here.

Things that remind me of Malawi sometimes set off in me a sort of posttraumatic stress reaction: hot, sticky days, certain odors, and diarrhea or fever in anyone in my family seem to hotwire my brain, bypassing higher-order thinking, reason, and the ability to form coherent narratives. I've heard British friends say "I'm losing the plot!" in the same way an American might say "I'm losing my mind," and that's about what it feels like: a few mosquito bites, a case of poison ivy, or a fever hardly spells doom when you live in New York, but my body and brain stem sometimes go into crisis mode at these times, ignoring what my prefrontal cortex has to say about the actual level of danger.

Despite the preventive measures deemed fanatical by most of our colleagues, our children got very sick in Malawi; Graeme had malaria at least twice, and once, it settled in his gut as gastric malaria, which I didn't even know existed; for at least a week he could barely keep in enough liquids to stave off dehydration. I brought him to the doctor everyday and debated whether or not to fly him to South Africa to be hospitalized, all while knowing that Malawian mothers buried children for lack of such luxuries. For a week I slept beside him and roused myself, and him, every ten minutes or so to give him a tiny sip of water.

That episode in Malawi activated earlier fears; four years before those long, hot nights of malarial fever, I lay on a hospital cot beside eighteen-month-old Graeme in a German university hospital. Through the thin mattress I could feel the bars of the frame, but I couldn't shift much, or I'd trouble the wires and tubes that connected him to monitors and IVs. The right side of his face was swollen and bruised. His right eye seemed weighted, and the weight of it rested on his right cheek, which hung low and jowly on his chin, and dragged down the right corner of his rosebud mouth. When I'd brought him to the emergency room, one young doctor took an accusatory tone: *tell me*, what has *happened* to your *child?* As if I had done this *to* him.

It started with a bit of a cold, a touch of a fever: nothing unusual for him. From the age of six months he had managed to catch every bug that made the rounds. During the gray, rainy Scottish winter, he got bronchitis. He got heatstroke in Rome and heatstroke in Paris. I was no stranger to the hospital and doctor's office, still, when I put Graeme down for a nap while Tim was studying in the other room, and went to the neighbors' for Sunday afternoon waffles and coffee, I didn't expect to return to find Graeme, still a baby in diapers and footie pajamas, looking as if he had been punched in the face, the soft semicircle under his right eye ballooned and ugly, red and blue.

I gathered a backpack—diapers, changes of clothes for him and for me, books for us both, an iPod, a water bottle, and some knitting—and called a taxi. Within the hour, they had admitted Graeme, started an IV of powerful antibiotics, and settled us in a room.

He would never sleep in the crib provided. He would sleep only in my arms, a feverish cherub with blond curls framing flushed cheeks, a doll of a baby whose grins drew the attentions of German grandmothers, who always wanted to know if he was a boy or a girl. The blond curls made it hard to tell.

"Ja, Mrs. Stone? The blood tells us there is a real infection!" The one nurse who knew enough English to speak with me was sent in. Yet not even she could tell me much more than that.

"Is he going to die?" I asked. She hesitated, and I couldn't discern why: Was she doing the mental gymnastics of translation? Or was she weighing how to tell me that death was a possibility. I asked again, "Is my son going to die?"

"No," she said. "He is not going to die."

But I could see in her eyes the reflection of myself, the near-hysterical mother, and her need to placate me, for it was very, very late by then. I crouched on the cot in the dark of the room, clutching my very sick baby in my arms, willing him to get well.

When my first son, Aidan, got his first cold, I couldn't shake the feeling of needing to blow my own nose each time I heard his snuffling inhalations; couldn't help clearing my own throat when his sounded clogged. When I noticed this, I thought: *I really* am *a mother now.*

"Mirror neurons!" my friend, a medical student, said.

Neuroscientists have described mirror neurons as one of their discipline's most significant discoveries in the last decade: brain scans suggest that mirror neurons respond to our observations of others, so that whether I'm in pain myself or observing someone who is, the map of my brain looks similar. It turns out that our brains are even great at reflecting the particular intensity of the pain that we are witnessing. The pictures of our brains outline the stories of our empathy.

When they jabbed the needle into Graeme to let the gut-scouring antibiotics flow into his blood, he cried, and so did I.

At least we didn't have to worry about whether or not our insurance would cover it. The doctors laughed when I expressed my worry over the cost of such a long hospital stay—"Oh, you are from America! Yes. Everything here insurance *must* cover." So we were spared that particular strain. But we had another child—Aidan, just four years old—and Tim was finishing his PhD research on a grant from the German government as well as preparing for job interviews (in a frightful economy) later that month. We had lived in Germany just two months, but immediately colleagues and acquaintances became friends—taking care of Aidan, bringing meals, visiting Graeme and me.

Graeme's face inflated even more with infection on the second and third day. I must have overheard the word *staph* because I remember the chill of that fear. I'd known of people dying from staph infections that started from a cat scratch or the nick of a razor. And a year earlier, while running through the streets of St. Andrews, Scotland, where we lived then, I had listened to a podcast on MRSA—methicillin-resistant staphylococcus aureus. MRSA (people just say it as if it were pronounced "mersa") is a staph infection that's resistant to almost every kind of existing antibiotic. The podcast—I have forgotten which one it was—compared the intractability of the virus to HIV and noted that annual deaths from MRSA were beginning to exceed those from AIDS.

The entwined barriers of language and culture held me back from panic as well as from asking what I wanted to know: *What kind of an infection did he have? What was the prognosis?* In the absence of facts, I imagined terrible things. I thought he might lose one of his sweet brown eyes. I imagined the infection traveling to his brain, since the brain isn't too far from the eye. I imagined multiple organ failure and ventilators. All the while I was unsure whether my fears were justified or based on my well-practiced habit of fearing— and bracing for—the very worst. My self-consciousness and pride in not wanting to be perceived as an overdramatic American before the stoic, serious, and intimidatingly good-looking German doctors held me back from maudlin display. I forced my face into something like composure while I listened to their explanations, which did little to dispel my ignorance, and when I left the room, I cried, or spent too much money calling my mom in New York.

One night in the hospital, I managed to get Graeme to sleep in his crib, took a shower, then wedged a chair in the doorway so I could knit by the light from the hallway. I was making fingerless gloves for Tim's sister. I had bought the wool in Rome, and it was detailed enough work that it took most of my attention. Needle in loop, thrown yarn, pull, repeat, reverse, knitting and purling, around and around, making just about the slowest progress possible. It may seem silly to manufacture that which can be so easily purchased, but I loved it. *What are you making?* a nurse whispered in German. *Fingerless mittens for my sister*, I said, because I didn't know how to say "sister in-law" in German. *Oh, they'll be good for bike riding, then*, the nurse said. *Yes*, I agreed, because I didn't know how to say *we don't ride bikes as transportation in most of America.* She said, *They're going to be beautiful.* I said, *Thank you very much.* That was about it, but it made me feel better just to speak a little with someone else, to make something with my hands while I waited for that storm to pass.

I marvel a little, now, at how I endured that time without the disencumbering effects of a pint of beer or a glass of wine or a half a tab of some nice benzodiazepine. A little over a year later, touched off by fears of unemployment, another broken leg, and a car accident, my anxiety became so bad—I would stop along the sidewalk and gasp in horror at a frightening thought—that my doctor prescribed something. But I weathered that particular storm without any such palliating substances. I lay long hours in that lumpy cot, holding my son, nursing him—it was the only nourishment he would take—and trying to breathe, breathing being the only kind of prayer, or almost-prayer, that I could manage. My theology didn't hold a lot of space for miracles, so I didn't pray for one; I just breathed in and out: *Lord, have mercy. Have mercy on me. This sea is so wide. My boat is so small. This sea is so wide. My boat is so small.* An Irish fisherman's prayer, or so I had heard, and one that puts me in mind of Moses' mother putting her tiny son in a tiny boat and casting him on the waters, hoping against hope that God, perhaps through the hands of some compassionate woman, will take him up again, deliver him.

This prayer also put me in mind of my childhood fear of water, and of the fear of all that is unknown below the surface of the sea, the fathomless depths with beasts both frightful and beautiful; both harmless and deadly. I felt like the psalmist:

> Save me, O God; for the waters are come in unto
> my soul.
> I sink in deep mire, where there is no standing;
> I am come into deep waters
> Where the floods overflow me. (Psalm 69:1-2 KJV)

Somewhere I heard this form of prayer or meditation suggested for difficult times: you imagine yourself on the top of a roiling sea—for that is what it feels like sometimes to live in this world full of worries. The water threatens to overwhelm the soul, the mind, the body even; you can't think clearly or sit still, you struggle even to swallow: anxiety feels like this, and it is awful. But even in awful times, even when the waves crest and fall and break over you, even when the surface is tempestuous and squally, far, far below the surface, where the whales sing, the water is still. You learn to live in the world, in its chaos and its sadness, but you let your anchor fall into the deep; far, far below the troubled surface of the waters.

I closed my eyes, feeling the churning waters in my soul. *God, be my anchor.* I waited for stillness, for the anchor to drop, for God to lead me to a rock higher than I, to separate the waters and make a dry path through them, to lead me beside still waters. When a stillness—not perfect stillness, but relative stillness—came over me, I at last faced the truth I had not wanted to accept: that in spite of everything, including my vigilant worry and care, my son could die. I had both given and sustained my sons' lives with my own body, had tried to sneeze and cough for them. Why had I never fully believed that my fierce love could not protect them, finally, from death? *When we are talking about mortality,* Joan Didion wrote, *we are always talking about our children.*

I really am a mother now.

I protect, I nourish, but in the very act of giving life I have relinquished control, or, better, realized the truth that control is an illusion. I do not want to demand my son's survival. I do not want to admit that his death is a possibility. To love is to unshield oneself—*shield* coming from a German word meaning "to separate"—and I was unshielded, unseparated, exposed, a fisherman caught in a storm in a dinghy on a churning sea. I tried to pray. If I had access to some substance that would numb, would separate me from the anxiety and the unknowing, I would have reached for it with both hands. Or would I? I held my boy in my arms, closed my eyes, and imagined an anchor slowly descending to the deep and holding there, and grace, our buoyancy, upraising us, holding us in the light.

Graeme remembers none of this, but he likes to hear the story. The plot is this: You were very sick. You were in the hospital. You had medicine going in through a needle in your arm. You made the man who mopped the hallways laugh with your mischievous grin. He called you his friend. You got well.

The late physician Paul Brand told a story about hearing a lecture by the famed anthropologist Margaret Mead. "What is the earliest sign of civilization?" she asked. Not tools, not agriculture, not even a clay pot—a healed femur, she said, holding one aloft. You never found healed bones in places where violence and competition abounded, where the fittest people's survival was the only law. There you might find skulls crushed by clubs or temples pierced by arrows. A healed femur, she said, implied that someone had cared for that person, presumably at some personal cost, until he or she was well and able again. Paul Brand thought of this when he studied boxes of bones collected from a monastery: five hundred years after the fact, "thin lines of healing" showed evidence of the monks' care, as telling and precious as any sacred writing.

Mercy and grace turn the plot, giving shape to the oldest and most beautiful thing in civilization: that human beings care for one another.

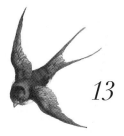

REFLECT

In several languages, including Italian and Spanish,

the word for birthmark means "cravings." In Dutch and

Danish, the term includes the word "mother," suggesting

that only one parent could be responsible for the spots.

OLGA KHAZAN, *"THE ODD SUPERSTITION BEHIND BIRTHMARKS"*

My great-grandmother Jennie, who bequeathed me the faulty gene for producing collagen, was killed by a drunk driver when my grandmother Charlotte was pregnant with my mom.

I've always liked the thought that part of me—or at least, the makings of the egg that would become part of me— resided in my mother before she was born, and that, therefore, in a sense, I, too, once resided inside my Grandma Charlotte: microscopic makings of a baby girl within a baby girl within a woman: a human matryoshka. I've wondered whether and how the shock of great-grandma Jennie's sudden death made an impression on my grandmother, and therefore, perhaps, on my not-yet-born mother, and even on me.

The theory of maternal impressions—the idea that what a woman sees or tastes or hears or touches or even *thinks* will imprint on her baby—is nearly universal in the catalog of traditional and prescientific beliefs. Increasingly, science suggests the grain of truth in the folk wisdom that what a pregnant woman sees, hears, or ingests will make an *impression* on the baby growing inside. Cultures from Italian to Hmong use the theory of maternal impressions to explain why a pregnant woman's cravings must be satisfied; if a pregnant woman craves strawberries and doesn't get any, her child will have a strawberry-shaped birthmark. Perversely, European cultures (and probably others) long believed that congenital disabilities were the result of the mother's evil sexual desires or sin. In the Massachusetts Bay Colony, Anne Hutchinson, the wealthy, wise woman (and sometime childbirth companion, including to Mary Dyer, the Quaker woman who was hung as a witch in 1660) who had come under scrutiny for her unorthodox religious teachings, delivered a large hyatidiform mole, which her detractors took to be a monster, a hideous incarnation of her repugnant teachings. A less perverse manifestation of the maternal impressions theory is the idea that if a mother is frightened by something while pregnant, her child will grow up to fear that same thing. And the idea that anxious mothers will give birth to anxious offspring is pretty much orthodox childbirth teaching, alas.

Following this theory, my grandmother's shock and grief and my great-grandmother's death may have impressed my mother with a fear of death by automobile accident, which she imparted to me. Grandma Charlotte never did earn her driver's license—not as a reaction to Jennie's death, exactly, but after dutifully attending driver's education, her instructor advised that it would be better for all concerned if she stuck to public transport. I was in third grade before my mother earned hers, and I didn't earn mine until age twenty-one—considerably older than my peers. I drive, but driving makes me anxious. I hate to let my children go somewhere in a car without me. I fret the minute that someone I care about is late. I perform internet searches for traffic accidents along the routes they may have taken. I fling myself upon my husband's neck when he returns from wherever, once again miraculously unharmed. From time to time, I gasp audibly, sometimes in public, because I've just vividly imagined someone I loved being killed with a car. Probably this has nothing whatever to do with Jennie. But so much of what is inherited is still uncharted water.

Perhaps somewhere, folded into whatever makes me this peculiar little person, I do carry some trace of fear about the specific means by which my great-grandmother died.

Following the Ashkenazi Jewish practice of naming for the one most recently deceased, my mother was given Jennie's name—Jeanette—and grew to look just like her, wide grin and twinkling eyes that a smile scrunches into half-moons: eyes that also bear the mark of OI. My eyes and my children's eyes also look like Jennie's.

When Jennie's second son, Bernie, was born, her spine collapsed. She could not care for my grandfather, Harold, and she placed him temporarily in an orphanage. From then on, Jennie was never able to straighten her back, was never not in physical pain. When Bernie was a toddler, Jennie tied one end of a rope around his waist and the other end around the tree in the front yard so he wouldn't run into the street and be killed by a car. She wouldn't have been able to move fast enough to save him. When Jennie became pregnant again, she had an abortion.

My grandmother told me this as we sat in a booth sipping our drinks—a ginger ale for me, a *vodka martini*

extra-extra-extra dry, up *with a twist* for her. She was un-apologetically prochoice and had encouraged my mom to have an abortion, later apologizing when I was born. (She brought a little sign to the hospital that said "Welcome to the World, Rachel Marie.")

For a long time, I did not know that as many as a fourth of women have abortions in the course of their lives. I was always ready to argue a prolife position, including, I'm ashamed to admit, that patent lie that a woman's body can't (or won't) conceive if she's raped—the politician who effectively ended his own campaign spouting such nonsense got that line from somewhere, just as I had. Someone brought little plastic fetus dolls representing babies at several different stages of prenatal development to our youth group; I held them in my hands, examining their fingers and eyelids. I had one of those tiny footprint-shaped lapel pins. I thought women who had abortions must be monsters. I thought my grandmother and great-grandmother must have been monsters.

To abort is to withhold consent to the blood sacrifice that every pregnancy exacts, or, perhaps, it is to exchange the mother's blood sacrifice in carrying the pregnancy to term for the fetus's blood sacrifice in being discarded as medical waste, or carefully dismembered and distributed for medical research. In no case is pregnancy ever bloodless. In no case does it eschew sacrifice of one kind or another.

Abortion is always a choice, and sometimes a choice between awful and less-awful: when a mother of four is dying of pulmonary edema and the only chance of saving her life is to abort her twelve-week pregnancy, when a nine-year-old child is raped by her father and becomes pregnant with twins, when a very poor woman knows she'll lose her job and be rejected by her family if she is found to be with child. Perhaps these are extreme examples, but perhaps not: rates of abortion correlate highly with poverty. Ideologues bicker. It is impossible, some say, to solve every social problem that would seem to make abortion a desirable or even necessary choice; ideologues on the other insist that abortion is nothing to be ashamed of or to regret or to try to prevent, as if it were no different than an appendectomy. Scholars of the history of reproduction say that whether legal or moral or otherwise, abortion has always been part of human experience, and studies demonstrate that making it illegal does little to reduce its prevalence. Birth control helps. Jennie, my great-grandmother, didn't have many options there, either.

I read somewhere that wild animals will sometimes spontaneously abort—that is, miscarry—if conditions are bad enough. If a new lion takes over the pride, for example, lionesses pregnant by another male will abort, knowing that the new lion will kill the cubs that aren't his as soon as they're born. Jennie's world was unaccommodating to people like her—an observant Jew living then in Tennessee, a woman with a disability. Her's was nearly a Sophie's choice: the choice between aborting the child in her womb so that she might go on mothering, albeit imperfectly and painfully, the children already born.

Catcalls and obscene attentions from strange men are sometimes how girls first realize that they're growing into women. My realization of womanhood came with my first transvaginal ultrasound, the kind that some state legislatures have proposed mandating for women seeking abortion, which I was not, though the pregnancy was a surprise. My obstetrician was less than encouraging. I have always looked young for my age, an attribute for which I was always told I would one day be grateful (and that day has come), but to appear sixteen and to be pregnant is to invite condescension. I endured the humiliations of invasive exams with my hands over my eyes. I obeyed the doctor when she made me meet with a genetic counselor who merely read back to me scary information I had already studied on my own. I let the doctor rush me through appointments and wave away my questions even as she labeled my pregnancy "high-risk" and scared me with stories of what might be. *If this is what it is to be a woman*, I thought during one embarrassing exam, *then I want out*. Sometimes being a woman means wanting, desperately, to escape from your body.

But I didn't have to worry about my spine collapsing like Jennie's. I had a titanium rod holding mine in place. When I was just seventeen, still living at home with my parents, I had an operation that kept me out of school for four months of my senior year. After the surgery, I took several pints of blood, contributed by friends from church who shared both my O+ blood type and my lingering, irrational HIV-fueled fear of New York blood banks. Before, as I slipped into the fog of anesthesia, my mother asked the surgeon to repeat the rationale for the surgery once more. I heard him say, *So she will stand straight*. I heard him say, *So she will be active into her old age*. I heard him say, *So she will play with her grandchildren*.

Three years earlier, my regular doctor spotted something in my posture that suggested asymmetry—though my posture, from years of ballet, was good—and ordered an X-ray. When the radiologist clipped it to the lightbox, I cringed. Nothing I had seen in the mirror had caused me to doubt that my spine was as tidily aligned as those belonging to the grinning skeletons diagrammed in medical books. Instead, the image of my insides was serpentine, an *S* curve well progressed, crooked, winding, not straight, in defiance of textbook spines. I saw in my deformed spine the embodiment of evil. I was diseased, marked with an *S* not just for scoliosis but for sin.

Orthopedic comes from two Greek words: *ortho*, meaning "straight" or "right," and *paideia*, meaning "rearing of children." Etymologically, to be an orthopedist is to specialize in raising kids right, which means raising them "straight" in all things skeletal. Like orthodontia, orthopedics is concerned with straightening what's crooked, bent, twisted, deformed. And like *orthodoxy*, which concerns itself with right or straight opinions (*doxa* = opinion) particularly in the area of theology, orthopedics aspires to conform the body to an external standard, an inflexible ideal.

My spine surgeon assured me that scoliosis had a preference for "smart, pretty girls" like me, but I was not fooled. The very name of my condition—adolescent idiopathic scoliosis—was awful. *Idiopathic* is just medical jargon for "we don't know what caused it" but stems from roots shared with words like *idiot* and *pathological*. I don't believe it was illogical for me to believe, as I did, that my scoliosis was a physical manifestation of some moral failing; as the word about my condition got around, I was regaled with tales of scoliosis "cured" through exercise, yoga, massage, and chiropractic, which gave the impression that straightening my spine would be a matter of applying due diligence and discipline, and not at all a question of inter-vertebral discs growing all wrong for no reason that anyone then could discern.

Some time before my diagnosis I had read a mawkish short story in an evangelical teen girls' magazine in which a high school student with scoliosis wore a brace that was, even by the time of that publication, very, very old-school: a con-traption of leather and foam and metal reaching up to and encircling the neck with a ring that had the look of some implement of torture. It had to be worn twenty-three hours a day, including the seven to ten most humiliating hours in a teenage girl's day: during school. All I can recall of the story is that the brace-wearing protagonist suffered mockery and discomfort, but that there was, I need hardly say, some im-portant spiritual lesson in it for her, some lesson that I most emphatically did not care to bone up on.

I too wore a brace for years, one that was required to be worn only at night. I imagined some empathetic innovator who understood that teenage girls tend to endure more than enough bodily mortification even without remedial encase-ments that look like something from the Spanish Inquisition. My brace was uncomfortable, but not embarrassing, since I wore it only in bed, and it was also entirely ineffective. I had to have the surgery anyway, a long, complicated surgery from which I awoke certain that I was dying.

Imagine sinking into nothingness, descending into utter blank, to a place where you are not, then slowly rising to awareness, to lurid brightness, to monitors that screech and to your own body's silent shrieking: flames licking the lining of your lungs and the back of your throat, consuming the engine of your very breath. You watch the huge wall clock and will yourself to plummet back below the surface and to stay there, in oblivion, for a long, long time, but the calm and starless intervals between periods of conscious pain are thirty seconds at most. In trying not to drown in the pain, you try not to fight it, for when you do fight it, you feel even worse. It takes all your strength to do what looks like nothing at all: to lie there and bear it, only appearing passive, but working harder than you ever have. Your eyes leak, salty tears running into the corners of your mouth; as in past humiliation, other people wash and dress you and tend to the private, necessary things you cannot take care of. You await the return of the sense that your body is a home, and not a prison. You hope that this perpetual labor will give birth to something in which you can rejoice.

Perhaps that labor did birth something to rejoice in. My spine is strong and has stayed strong, and I gave birth, twice, as vigorously as the daughters of Israel whose fertility could not be stayed by Pharaoh's murderous decree. I have carried my children in my womb and on my back and in my arms, and I stand straight still. Jennie's misery was never mine. I never had to tie one of my children to a tree or give them into the care of others or flush one from my womb. I have been fortunate. I have not been alone, bent and broken, trying to bear an unbearable burden.

One night in New York, when our children were small, a drunk driver in a truck jumped the curb, ran through our front yard, uprooting trees as it went, and crashed through the wall of the church next door. *Thank God no one was in the yard; thank God he missed the house and ran into the empty church; thank God, thank God.* For more than a year, I flinched at passing vehicles and panicked when my kids played outside. When even deep breathing and logical thinking could not stop my panic, my doctor wrote a prescription for anti-anxiety medicine. I thought of Jennie, the woman who had cradled baby Elise's lifeless body; Jennie, killed by a drunk driver when my mom, with the makings of me inside her, was nestled inside Charlotte, my grandma. My mom was there, and part of me was there, when Charlotte sat shiva, tossed shovels full of dirt on plain pine boxes for mother and for daughter, and wept.

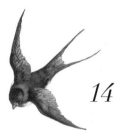

GROAN

After a good dinner one can forgive anybody,

even one's own relatives.

OSCAR WILDE

In Malawi, I often saw my neighbor Dahlia sitting outside with her daughters and another woman or two. They would unroll hand-woven straw mats and make themselves comfortable in the shade. On one very hot day, I saw Dahlia's friend—or maybe her cousin—braiding Dahlia's hair. I sat down with them for a moment. Dahlia smiled in greeting from the corners of her eyes so as not to disturb the patient, painstaking transformation of her hair into tiny rows of intricate plaits. It would take hours. They would talk or sit

in companionable silence, and though I was always wel-
comed warmly, I could feel the disruption of my presence—
the embarrassment of the young cousin who could not speak
English well, the straining for topics of conversation—and I
never stayed long.

When we were young, my godsister Sarah—my mother is
her godmother and hers is mine, so we declared ourselves
"godsisters" when we were very young—loved to do my hair.
Or maybe she didn't love it, but felt that it should be done.
My hair has been more or less of a mess my whole life, and
Sarah was always tidying it up. She'd sit me in front of a
mirror, and I'd watch her face grow serious as she worked a
comb through the tangles, slick down frizz with water and
a swipe of gel, and set to work divvying my hair into pairs
of French braids so tight that they raised my eyebrows. If I
wiggled during a crucial maneuvering of the hair, she'd slap
the side of my head and hiss *Don't. Move.* I adored every
minute of it. I worshiped Sarah.

In Malawi I was lonely for the company of women, so
lonely, in fact, that I thought about paying one of the women
at the little beauty stalls in the open-air market to braid my
hair, just for the feeling of closeness, something approxi-
mating friendship. The market was loud and hot and full of
strong smells, and even as I longed for connection, my
worries about germs prevailed, so I stayed home, cut my own

hair (badly), braided it as best I could and, lacking a second mirror to check the back, took pictures of the back of my head with my phone.

I don't mind being alone. I like it and need it. But women in Malawi seemed rarely to be alone, and my own loneliness was a source of shame to me there. A friend once told me that if a Malawian sees a person walking or sitting alone, they assume that the person is sad or unwell. Their way of being in constant, close contact with friends and relatives is certainly more common, historically and globally, and though I wouldn't dare romanticize what it means to be born a woman in many traditional societies, deep woman-to-woman friendships and a sense of female solidarity and community seems to be something that most women long for and read for, particularly as they become mothers. In the absence of crowds of mothers and mothers-in-law and aunts and sisters and female cousins, those in industrialized countries reach for parenting books and professionals who can tell us what to expect from our pregnancies, from our newborns, from our toddlers. With the ever-present internet and social media, we can, with a few taps of the screen, pose our questions to hundreds or thousands of people, many of whom will be willing to dispense advice while denouncing the advice of others, setting off skirmishes in what's known, belittlingly, as the "Mommy Wars."

Perhaps my great-grandma Katherine—called Kitty—would have ignited a "Mommy War" controversy over her decision to give birth to my Grandma Peggy at home, with a doctor in attendance. It was 1928, and by then, most births in New York City took place in hospitals. But Kitty had heard that the hospital food was no good. Still, home births were common enough—and close enough to everyone's memory—that it was likely regarded as a respectable choice. That was also the year that Alexander Fleming discovered the mold that eventually made penicillin, but at the time of my grandmother's birth, antibiotics didn't exist, and avoiding hospitals as much as possible made a certain kind of sense—as it does to many people today, in the age of antibiotic-resistant microbes. Before sulfa drugs and antibiotics, and especially before the germ theory of disease was understood, the main killer of childbearing women was puerperal fever (also called "childbed fever"), which was a strep or staph or E. coli infection of the recently vacated and therefore highly tender womb. Though cases of childbed fever are documented in ancient Greek literature as early as the fifth century BCE, it became increasingly common as most births moved from home to hospital. The diaries of the informally trained Maine midwife Martha Ballard, which she kept from 1785 to 1812, show an impressive survival rate: the women she assisted in childbirth fared six times better than women giving birth in hospitals in London and Dublin.

The first teaching hospital in the world was Paris's Hôtel-Dieu (literally, God's Hotel). It is also the oldest hospital that is still functioning. In its early years, poor and indigent women were encouraged to give birth there in part so that their bodies could serve as "teaching material" to doctors in training. That they died in such large numbers was attributed to God's judgment on their immoral lifestyles—not to the dirty hands of the physicians and students, who moved between patients, and even between autopsies of ex-patients in the morgue, without washing their hands. It was hard for people to imagine that a person of "good moral character," like a medical doctor, could be the source of the scourge (assigning moral import to illness did not begin during the AIDS crisis), but it was true. The very high rates of childbed death in some European hospitals—one observer noted that a woman who gave birth in the street, literally, was better off than a woman in a hospital—had a way of impressing the imagination, however, and people came to regard childbirth as inherently dangerous, and, perhaps ironically, safest when done in the hospital.

My great-grandma Kitty was no stranger to illness. She'd nearly died ten years earlier when she contracted the dreaded and deadly influenza of 1918, which wiped out as many as 6 percent of all people living on earth in a single year. It killed people of her age—late teens—especially. Most strains of flu sweep away the very old and the very young, but the 1918 flu had a penchant for people in young adulthood. It laid her low for a year, but she got better, thus prompting the belief, handed down through the generations, that she, and therefore *we*, were of "hardy stock." She advised such treatments for illness as wrapping your chest in a woolen scarf, staying in bed, and drinking hot toddies made with Christian Brothers' brandy.

Kitty was one of the three great-grandmothers still living when I was small. There's a small snapshot of the two of us flanking my father. I'm sitting in a stroller in a sundress, looking at her and Chloe, her dog, some kind of German shepherd mutt much like my own German shepherd mutt from Malawi. I remember being afraid of Chloe. I remember that Kitty seemed very old and very tall, and that I didn't know how to react when my parents told me she'd died. She was moody and temperamental, a worrier—the same woman who built a beach house and then fretted about tracking in sand. I feel that she and I would have understood one another completely, and this worries me too.

Like her, I hate going places where the food is no good, and if I had to eat thirty meals of hospital food—women in those days stayed about ten days after childbirth—I'd be looking for alternatives, too, because the hunger that follows labor and delivery is a righteous and overpowering hunger, and breastfeeding only enhances it. The old wives' tale says that a woman loses a tooth for every child she bears—a reality still in many pockets of the world—which points to the great demand on a woman's store of calcium and minerals and nutrients. The midwives in Malawi told me that pica—the overwhelming urge to chew and eat nonfood items (coal, dirt, cloth)—is pretty common. I suppressed a gasp once while visiting a rural birth center when a young woman holding her new baby grinned at me, showing gums white with anemia. I'd first begun caring about global maternal health when, pregnant with my second child, I happened upon the blog of an American midwife in Malawi. While I was eager to ingest the ideal proportions of fatty acids to aid the development of optimal intelligence in my unborn baby, other women were dying in the birthing bed for lack of the most basic nutrients.

Though I was never unusually hungry during pregnancy—my torso was too short to allow my stomach much room for expansion—the hunger afterward was tremendous. I ate chocolate bars and bananas and drank milk in the middle of the night, with animal urgency. We bought these things in bulk at Costco, and my husband took to setting out snacks by my bedside table before retiring himself, knowing that both baby and I would wake up desperate for nourishment. A woman from church brought us a perfect meal on a tray with flowers, and I wept with gratitude. She understood that the hunger of new motherhood is not merely physical but a hunger for beauty and graciousness, that in those early days you wonder if your eating will ever lose its newfound feral quality, whether you will ever get out of your pajamas again, and whether you will ever again eat a full meal, at a table, using both your hands.

Far from being frivolous, then, my great-grandma Kitty's concern over what she'd be eating postpartum had deep and respectable roots. In early America, childbirth was a social event; most women, writes Laurel Thatcher Ulrich, "literally gave birth in the arms or on the laps of their neighbors." The midwife herself might check in with the mother in early labor, but when things got serious, it was time for the "calling of the women," who arranged to help the mother with her household duties—most of which related in some way to the preparation of food—until she was ready to return to the kitchen. Martha notes in her diary after one birth that "the ladies who assisted took supper after all our matters were completed," and it has the ring of a celebration. Elsewhere, early American women wrote of the "groaning table"—a meal that a newly delivered mother would offer to her friends in thanks and celebration after her period of "lying-in" was completed and she returned to her regular activities. The word *groaning* poked fun at the noises women make during labor and also highlighted the abundance of the feast, which (in good years) was plentiful enough to make the table groan under the weight of it all. The British anthropologist Sheila Kitzinger claims that the happy female socialization buzzing around births aroused male contempt; the word *gossip*, she says, comes from the word *godsibs*—god siblings: the bond of sisterhood forged in the fire of labor.

I gave birth to my second son in a Scottish hospital, where tradition demands that a tray of tea and toast be brought in as soon as a woman delivers. It wasn't *my* tradition, but the elements of the ritual were familiar enough so that nothing could have been more delicious or more comforting just then. My great-grandmother, in choosing to give birth at home, where her mother could care for her, and where she could eat her own food, must have understood the significance of that comfort, much as the women in Martha Ballard's community did. In her deeply empathetic study of one family's struggle navigating the ideological chasm between their ancient traditional culture and contemporary American medical culture, Anne Fadiman notes that Hmong culture prescribes a specific postpartum menu of steamed rice and chicken boiled with five special herbs. The father in her story, Nao Kao, grew these herbs in one corner of his apartment complex's parking lot in Northern California, cooked the traditional meal, and brought it to his wife, Foua, as she recovered in the hospital after her fifth child was born while Foua was "lying on her back on a steel table"— in contrast to how their older children had been born: into Foua's own hands, in a dirt-floored home in the Old Country. Foua was willing to submit to what must have seemed to her the strange indignities of a hospital birth, but having the right sort of food afterward was nonnegotiable, necessary to her complete recuperation. Who hasn't known this—the comfort of familiar food in difficult or painful times?

After my second son was born, we took him home from the Scottish hospital to the small university town where we lived, which might have been the setting of a storybook. It lies between the farmlands and the sea, and the town's streets still follow their medieval layout, stretching from their common source, the cathedral where St. Rule is rumored to have brought the relics of St. Andrew to rest thousands of years ago. The ruins of a castle stand nearby, and on Sundays, anyone at all can stroll the immaculate and gently rolling greens of the Old Course, the oldest golf course in the world, while the North Sea laps the beach just below. The town is small enough that few of the American student families who lived there owned (or needed) cars, and we enjoyed a cozy proximity, meeting for book clubs and at church, but also informally as we passed in shops or the library. Because so many babies were being born, and so many of us were so far from home, the tradition of bringing meals to families with new babies developed: a meal every other night for a month. Sometimes I rolled my eyes when yet another email went out asking for volunteers to make meals, but when my turn came, it was a true gift. Lasagna, casseroles, salad, brownies, stew and stir-fry—sacraments of love: outward and visible signs of inward and spiritual grace. These meals were the sustaining body and blood of Christ, given because God so loves the world—*this world!*—that God is making it new by a love that leads to wholeness, which is, after all, another way of saying *holiness*, and which comes to us, often, through food that is delicious and nourishing, prepared and offered with love from one human being to another. The bread and the wine. The casserole and the salad. The eucharistic table and the groaning table.

In hospitals, the farmer-poet Wendell Berry has written,

Food is treated as another unpleasant substance to inject. And this is a shame. For in addition to the obvious nutritional link between food and health, food can be a pleasure. . . . Mealtimes offer three opportunities a day when patients could easily be offered something to look forward to. Nothing is more pleasing or heartening than a plate of nourishing, tasty, beautiful food artfully and lovingly prepared.

Even if the state of food in most hospitals does far fall from any ideal, whether aesthetic, nutritional, or spiritual, most of us do go there to have our babies. Some will choose, as my great-grandmother did, to stay at home to give birth, and it sometimes feels easy to label such choices as frivolous or dangerous, simply because we do not comprehend all that is implied in such a choice.

In a world as globally networked as ours, it's not unusual to find oneself traversing the jagged borders between competing—or even apparently conflicting—views of the world. What does not seem to change is that women, in every place and at every time, need to feel safe and comfortable wherever they choose to give birth, and, when they have done so, to be nourished; nourished with food that is not only good to eat but, as the French anthropologist Claude Lévi-Strauss said, "good to *think*," food that comforts us because it has been offered with love because it conforms to a menu that's traditional and familiar, or because it evokes some kind of nostalgia—that *nostos algos* or "home pain," that longing for something we can no longer quite access, that feeling of identification with family or community or traditions long lost. Why do I *want* to know the ways in which I might resemble my foremothers? Perhaps because we all want to know where we belong and with whom. And perhaps food whispers that to us, tangibly, intimately.

The house where my grandmother was born still stands, or did, the last time anyone looked, though the name of the street was changed. The thought is strangely comforting, even though I've never seen it and probably never will. But I like knowing it's there. It's a reminder that there are people to whom I belong, and we all need people whose hands we welcome when they brush our hair or bring us food, and perhaps never more than when we are, or have just finished, groaning.

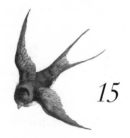

TILL WE
BECOME REAL

Holy places are dark places. It is life and strength,

not knowledge and words, that we get in them. Holy wisdom

is not clear and thin like water, but thick and dark like blood.

C. S. LEWIS, *TILL WE HAVE FACES*

I walked to the clinic and asked for the HIV test. The technician drew blood and tested it while I waited in the hall. After a few minutes he handed me a slip of paper with a number 10 written on it. Then the doctor called me in and took my slip of paper.

"Negative!" he boomed, smiling.

"Then why is there a 10?" I asked.

"We use a code to prevent people reading their own test results."

But I had to come back for another test, just to be certain, in a few weeks. Again I waited, received my slip of paper (this time, it was folded) and peeked in while I waited. *10*. But what if they'd changed the code, and 10 now meant "positive"? The clinician—no doctor in the house today—called me in.

"Negative."

I let out a whoop and high fived him.

My chance of being infected was never high. Every day, my chances of contracting some other potentially fatal illness—or dying in a car crash—were far higher than my chance of acquiring HIV from the blood and water of a stranger's womb. But anxiety often feels easier to manage if it is focused on something specific: HIV, cancer, refugees, people who are homeless or who look different than we do. It is irrational and dangerous, and it is how many of us live without realizing what we're doing. Still, in Malawi, some risks were real, and for whatever reason, one or more members of our family seemed always to be sick: malaria, giardia, chronic respiratory infections, and nameless fevers.

And there was sickness in our community there, too: infighting and gossip and allegations of sexual harassment and financial malfeasance. Tim and I did what we could, and then we gave up. We bought tickets, put a date on the calendar, sold off our furniture, and tried to help our housekeeper find another job. I paid a man to help me get an export permit for the dog, since, having kept her alive for nearly a year, I wasn't about to give her up. She might, like other dogs there, end up penned in a concrete block and half-starved all day and urged to run wild and vicious all night. We got on a plane with the dog, and then another, and then, impossible though it seemed, we were in New York. For weeks I luxuriated in the sense that all my preoccupying fears were suddenly irrelevant. We could eat raw fruits and vegetables without washing them in bleach. I could rinse my toothbrush with tap water. When my kids got mosquito bites, they itched, but they did not come down with infectious diseases. I whispered to myself: *Remember how wonderful this is, this feeling of being home and safe at last. Try to stay unworried. Be thrilled by raw vegetables forever.*

I knew, in time, that I would dream up new things to be anxious about, that I would acclimate quickly to the ordinary luxury of America, and that life itself would keep giving me actual challenges to face, starting with (once again) moving, and setting up a new home—*again.*

For a while, and even now, when I think of the many hot and sticky and sick, anxious, tearful days in Malawi, I think of the biblical metaphor of being in prolonged labor only to give birth to wind. But there is a crack in the vessel in which I placed that story—Mark, our dearest student. Before we left, we gave him stacks of books, notebooks and pens, and a solar-powered lantern for reading after dark. He was unusual among his peers in that he constantly read, well beyond what was assigned, and I felt toward him as I might have felt toward a younger brother, if I'd had one: proud and admiring and ever so slightly maternal. We shared news over email, and once he wrote this: *I always remember your family for your friendliness to me. Friends are a family God grants us. You are part of my family.* So there was this. Perhaps, I thought, Malawi had not been a miscarriage after all.

The Sunday after that email was Pentecost—when churches remember the Holy Spirit descending on the first followers of Jesus, allowing them to speak in many different languages. The priest invited a guest to read one of the Scripture portions, and introduced him as a clergyman visiting from Malawi. I marched up to him during the passing of the peace and, extending my right hand with my left hand resting on my right forearm, I greeted him in Chichewa. His eyes widened with the surprise of hearing his own language in a foreign city, eight thousand miles from home. After the benediction we talked, quickly narrowing in on people in Malawi we both knew. *Did you know that Dahlia was in the hospital?* he asked. *Yes, her nephew told me,* I said.

Small world, the church people said. *Small world.*

My grandma Peggy lived long enough to be relieved when we came back from Malawi. Ebola exploded in West Africa just as we were leaving, and though it was thousands of miles away from Malawi, she, like lots of people, felt better once we left the continent entirely. Not long after, she died. She lived out the last ten or so years of her life at the beach house in East Hampton, but I am fairly certain that she made it through her last decade without enjoying her beautiful surroundings much, though she did have to weather a few hurricanes and superstorms in the gymnasium of the local high school. She refused to let my dad come evacuate her; she worried something would happen to him on the way. It's an anxiety I recognize.

I always knew the beach house would be sold when she died. It was what she wanted, and it made sense. When Kitty built the house, the landscape was all the riches anyone needed, and the homes were humble, mere shelter at the end of a day spent outdoors. All around the little beach house now were palaces with high hedgerows and manicured lawns, many owned by corporations and celebrities. The little cluster of cottages on the dune was now a place to see and be seen. As much as I wanted to hold on to that place, times had changed and so had the place, and it was time to let go.

Still, that last summer I made sure that my sons went to the beach house with my dad. He showed them all the places he played when he was small and told them stories about the families whose houses were there, and there, and there: how they'd take off their shoes at the end of June, upon arriving, wincing and ouching their way across hot sand and rocky paths, and how, by the end of August, their feet were brown and leathery. Aidan and Graeme insisted on going barefoot, too. My mom texted me a picture—the three of them, flip-flops in hand, walking down the road to the ocean.

My younger son, Graeme, often talks about death. Like me, he zeros in on the bird that can't fly, the stray cat that's starving and limping, or the squashed bunny on the side of the road. When I was a child, I took these things in and said nothing, holding in sadness like a cough I didn't want to release, lying awake at night thinking of a baby turtle I'd seen flattened like a bottle cap on the blacktop. But Graeme has an openness I never did. He'll cry openly, talk about what is bothering him, and announce his delight in unself-conscious detail: "I love to eat a whole little tomato and feel it *pop* and feel how the seeds just *burst* through your mouth." One Saturday morning, he climbed into my lap and asked, "How will I be able to *find* you in heaven?" When I hesitated, his chin wobbled.

"Listen," I said. "Listen. I don't understand everything in the Bible, but it does say this—'love is stronger than death.' I will *always* find you."

The children's book *The Velveteen Rabbit* is sometimes invoked as a semi-Christian parable—the idea is that love is what makes you real; in the book, a toy bunny that's loved so hard that he's threadbare is sent out to be burned after the little boy who loved him gets scarlet fever. Because the bunny may be a disease vector, he's got to go. As he cries in the garden, awaiting his fate, the Nursery Magic Fairy comes and turns him into a real bunny. He joins the other bunnies, and the next spring, the boy, now recovered, spots the bunny in the garden and thinks he sees a resemblance to his old velveteen rabbit. This is supposed to be heartwarming, but I've never been able to stomach it—I regard it as unbearably sad. If being real and resurrected makes you unrecognizable to the ones you love the most, what good is it? To me, the story is anything but comforting.

I thought about this as I held Graeme that morning. He put his head on my chest, and I prayed silently that I would be able to keep my promise—that one day, long from now, he would open his eyes in a world like this one, better, but recognizable, and find out what it is to have all that has been lost restored. Once I heard the Israeli poet Rivka Miriam say of the people in her land, "we are in permanent labor, and we don't know what kind of baby we are giving birth to." She was talking about the future of her nation-state, but it had the ring of universal truth. What comes at the end of this life, full of struggles large and small? St. Paul says that the whole creation, including us, groans as if in childbirth, waiting to see what kind of redemption awaits us; what there may yet be.

I hope that the life of the world to come is as surprising as a new baby when it first emerges to the light—the verb, in Spanish, "to give birth" is *to give to the light*. You know that a baby is coming, and you may know that it is a boy or a girl, and you may know something about what it looks like, but even if you know all this, even if you have carried it within your own body for months and months, it is both as familiar and as strange as any stranger could be, far more helpless than a baby deer. But you are not in any doubt about to whom this baby belongs. You recognize her.

The vision of John in the book of Revelation says that God will wipe away every tear, and I hope that is true for sweat, too, for there is no shortage of either in the process of giving birth, whether to babies or to art to ideas or to salvation or to anything else. I hope we remember that so much of life involves struggle, and to numb ourselves for all the hard parts is to cease to live—and maybe, even, to sleep through the joy that comes in the morning. I hope that we remember that though we are each born naked and alone, trapped inside the subjectivity of our own person, the borders of our own skin, we can learn to belong to one another. We can risk contamination, can touch hands, can share. I hope we will remember that there will always be risk in whatever we do or don't do.

I hope *I* will remember.

"Life is just . . . all of that *and* all of *that*!" I said to Tim. On a walk down to the lake I had seen an amazing thing: a baby mallard being fostered by a pair of Canada geese. It was beautiful, this interspecies adoption, and it gave me hope. *There is kindness and hospitality, even in the animal world,* I thought. Then, on the walk back, I had seen a fledgling sparrow fallen from the nest, crushed on the sidewalk. Life is all of that *and* all of that. The sweet and the bitter. The sorrow and the joy.

I went to the beach house too, one last time, with my boys and my mom. I wandered through the rooms, touching things, crying a little. My aunt gave me some things: a rosary, a shot glass, a quilt made by my great-grandmother, an enamel chamber pot that my great-grandmother Kitty had used throughout her year of being bedridden with influenza. Tim thinks it is ridiculous that I wanted it, but I think it's a symbol of survival and resilience. I think I'm going to plant it full of succulents.

Each night at the beach house, Graeme and I squeezed into a single twin bed (he was small enough still, but surely not for long), and I smelled the salt in his hair and skin as we fell asleep listening to the waves and the wind in the dunes through the wide-open windows. Each day we ate lunch early and headed to the beach for the afternoon. I told them about that rotten, stinky whale, and secretly hoped we'd see another. My mother and I settled our beach chairs into the sand and talked and talked, mending old hurts, knitting new bonds, trying to do better. Again and again we hold out the hope of continuing to grow, continuing to change, continuing to hope that all will be well, that all will be *better*. That we will keep holding one another in the light.

Graeme came up from the water, that last day, and sat next to me on the rainbow quilt we've always used as a beach blanket. My mom went up the beach with Aidan to look for a lost toy. "We should be grateful for Grandma," Graeme said out of the silence. "We should be grateful for her because we wouldn't exist without her."

"Yes," I said. "That's true."

His brother came back, and they ran for the water once again. My mother sat back down. "Come on," I said. "Let's go in, too."

"I'm scared!" she said, but she got up.

The four of us joined hands and ran into the surf together, and then looked beyond the billows to the calm, wide sea. It went on and on for what looked like forever.

Faith should give us buoyancy, my pastor said in her sermon one Sunday. *Think about the way water holds you. It doesn't constrict you. You have freedom. Certain constraints, yes, but freedom to frolic. Our life in God is like that.*

We left the beach house for the last time, and took with us some old bodyboards from the shed. "You're going to let them go out on those?" my mother asked.

"Sure I am," I said. "If they want to."

It's not that I wasn't nervous. I was almost never not nervous that summer. But that day, I reclined on my rainbow quilt as my boys ran for the water with their boards, paddling fearlessly over the surface of the water as it grew deeper, as the waves caught them up and carried them on and on, and the sun sparkled on the surface of the water like thousands of diamonds, present for just a moment; impossible to grasp.

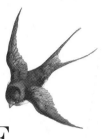

GRATITUDE

Many people—editors, writing colleagues, friends—read portions of this book in various forms. You know who you are. Thank you.

Amy Julia Becker and Katherine Willis Pershey workshopped many chapters with me; Ellen Painter Dollar, Kerri Fisher, Chris Park, Andrew Troutman-Taylor, and Lauren Winner all read much larger and more unwieldy versions. All of you offered helpful comments. Thank you.

I am grateful to the Collegeville Institute for twice hosting me and providing nourishment, shelter, and space for writing. Particular thanks goes to Don Ottenhof and Carla Durand.

As ever, I am grateful to my sons, Graeme and Aidan, and to my husband, Tim, for their unflagging support and love. (But it is your existence I love you for, mainly.)

NOTES

1 FLOAT

10   *I have read that a woman's body acquires*: Carl Zimmer, "The Cords That Aren't Cut," *New York Times*, September 15, 2015, D3.

3 REFLECT

33   *Recent studies in genetics*: See Aaron Kase, "Science Is Proving Some Memories Are Passed Down from Our Ancestors," Reset.me, February 20, 2015, http://reset.me/story/science-proving-memories -passed-ancestors.

5 DIVE

53   *In 1591, Agnes Sampson*: David Harley, "Historians as Demonologists: The Myth of the Midwife-Witch," in *Childbirth: Midwifery Theory and Practice*, ed. Philip K. Wilson (London: Routledge, 1996), 14.

        The nineteenth-century poet Julia Ward Howe: Elaine Showalter, *The Civil Wars of Julia Ward Howe: A Biography* (New York: Simon & Schuster, 2016), 86.

58   *rates of medical induction of labor*: Michelle J. K. Osterman and Joyce A. Martin, "Recent Declines in Induction of Labor by Gestational Age," National Center for Health Statistics, Centers for Disease Control and Prevention, June 2014, www.cdc.gov/nchs/products /databriefs/db155.htm.

61   *The philosopher Elaine Scarry*: Elaine Scarry, *The Body in Pain: The Making and Unmaking of the World* (New York: Oxford University Press, 1987), 11.

Pain has an element of blank: Emily Dickinson, Poem 650, in *The Complete Poems of Emily Dickinson*, ed. Thomas H. Johnson (Boston: Back Bay Books, 1960).

63 *Among the prolific writings*: Cotton Mather, *Elizabeth in Her Holy Retirement* (Boston: B. Green, 1710), pamphlet. Original spelling and punctuation retained.

He had a firebomb tossed through his window: Eula Biss, *On Immunity: An Inoculation* (Minneapolis: Graywolf Press, 2014).

64 *rates of maternal mortality*: "Maternal Mortality," US Department of Health and Human Services, Health Resources and Services Administration, https://mchb.hrsa.gov/whusa10/hstat/mh/pages /237mm.html.

65 *to suffer unnecessarily is masochistic*: Viktor Frankl, *Man's Search for Meaning* (Boston: Beacon Press, 2006), 113.

66 *far from wanting to be rescued*: Adrienne Rich, *Of Woman Born: Motherhood as Identity and Experience* (New York: Norton, 1995), 158. See also the edited transcript of Audre Lord in conversation with Adrienne Rich on the subject. She quotes her own poem: "How much of this truth can I bear to see and still live unblinded? How much of this pain can I use?" Audre Lord, *Sister Outsider: Essays and Speeches* (New York: Crossing Press, 2007), 106.

6 MOTHER

68 *No human creature could receive*: Dorothy Day, *The Long Loneliness* (New York: HarperOne, 2009), 139.

The lower animals: Wendell Berry, "The Peace of Wild Things," in *The Selected Poems of Wendell Berry* (Berkeley, CA: Counterpoint, 1999), 30.

72 *The humorist Mallory Ortberg*: Mallory Ortberg, "Leaving, Loving, and Laughing at the Church," talk at the Festival of Faith and Writing, Calvin College, 2016.

74 *One of the most astonishing*: Kathleen Norris, *The Cloister Walk* (New York: Riverhead Books, 1996), 24.

75 *Trible identifies the love*: Phyllis Trible, *God and the Rhetoric of Sexuality* (Minneapolis: Fortress Press, 1986), 33, 38.

77　*My Charley*: Harriet Beecher Stowe, *Life of Harriet Beecher Stowe*, compiled by Charles Edward Stowe (New York: Houghton, Mifflin, 1889), 126.

7 BAPTIZE

82　*Birth itself induces Pharaoh's hate*: Many of my observations in this section have been generally informed by the section "Exodus" in *Women's Bible Commentary*, ed. Carol A. Newsom and Sharon Ringe, exp. ed. with Apocrypha (Louisville: Westminster John Knox, 1998), esp. 33-44.

84　*Narrow was the passageway*: Tikva Frymer-Kensky, *Motherprayer: The Pregnant Woman's Spiritual Companion* (New York: Riverhead Books, 1995).

88　*Christians use the image of God as a warrior*: L. Julianna M. Claassens argues that while warrior images for God were appropriate for the nation of Israel—a small, beleaguered people among more powerful nations—it is less fitting in contexts such as the United States, which is already so culturally and militarily powerful and influential. In the United States, she suggests, people need to hear more about God's delivering presence in feminine and nonviolent terms. L. Julianna M. Claassens, *Mourner, Mother, Midwife: Reimagining God's Delivering Presence in the Old Testament* (Louisville, KY: Westminster John Knox, 2012).

　　The book of Isaiah: See Isaiah 42. See also Lauren F. Winner, "Laboring Woman," in *Wearing God: Clothing, Laughter, Fire, and Other Overlooked Ways of Meeting God* (New York: Harper One, 2015).

8 VESSEL

92　*And though the World Health Organization*: "Schistosomiasis," World Health Organization, accessed September 1, 2017, www.who.int /schistosomiasis/en.

93　*Insecticide-treated bed nets*: Jeffrey Gettleman, "Meant to Keep Malaria Out, Nets Are Used to Haul Fish In," *New York Times*, January 25, 2015, A1.

102　*the power and powerlessness embodied*: Adrienne Rich, *Of Woman Born: Motherhood as Identity and Experience* (New York: Norton, 1995), 96.

10 BAPTIZE

124 *For some, the phrase carries a whiff*: Rosemary Radford Ruether, *Sexism and God Talk* (Boston: Beacon Press, 1993), 246.

which is why midwives: See, for example, Heinrich Kramer and James Sprenger, *Malleus Maleficarum* [Hammer of Witches] (1486). This famous witch hunt manual singled out midwives as objects of particular scorn. This book, readable in English translation online, is discussed and quoted in Barbara Ehrenreich and Deirdre English, *Witches, Midwives, and Nurses: A History of Women Healers*, 2nd ed. (New York: Feminist Press at CUNY, 2010), and Barbara Ehrenreich, *For Her Own Good: Two Centuries of the Experts' Advice to Women*, 2nd ed. (New York: Anchor Books, 2005).

Because of this communication: Nicolas Malebranche, in *Malebranche: The Search After Truth*, ed. Thomas M. Lennon and Paul Olscamp, Cambridge Texts in the History of Philosophy (New York: Cambridge University Press, 1997), 600.

125 *"Reason," claims the philosopher*: Sara Ruddick, *Maternal Thinking: Towards a Politics of Peace* (Boston: Beacon Press, 1989), 194-95.

Catholic teaching officially: Catechism of the Council of Trent, part 1: The Creed, article 3.

The second-century apocryphal Gospel: Also known as the *Infancy Gospel of James*. A full translated text can be found at www.asu.edu /courses/rel376/total-readings/james.pdf.

126 *Addressing Mary herself*: The *Sermone de Navitate* (Nativity Sermon) attributed to St. Augustine is quoted by St. Thomas Aquinas in the *Summa Theologica*, Q35.A2, which can be found at the Christian Classics Ethereal Library, www.ccel.org/ccel/aquinas/summa.TP_ Q35_A6.html.

129 *Obedience is not a virtue*: Tikva Frymer-Kensky, *Motherprayer: A Pregnant Woman's Spiritual Companion* (New York: Riverhead Trade, 1996), 39.

133 *a meek and simple maid*: Julian of Norwich, *Revelations of Divine Love (Short Text and Long Text)* (New York: Penguin Books, 1998), 8.

135 *This is the miracle that saves the world*: Hannah Arendt, quoted in Ruddick, *Maternal Thinking*, 209.

135 *[He] was in labor*: Julian of Norwich, *Revelations of Divine Love*, 141.

136 *Wholeness*: Ruddick, *Maternal Thinking*, 215.

12 DIVE

146 *Dunning, a notorious Chicago asylum*: Robert Loerzel, "The Story of Dunning, A 'Tomb for the Living,'" *Curious City*, WBEZ Chicago, April 30, 2013, www.wbez.org/shows/curious-city/the-story-of -dunning-a-tomb-for-the-living/6d71dc74-bb21-4a25-8980 -c2d7a5670b06.

infant mortality rates: "Vital Statistics of the United States: 1890-1938," National Center for Health Statistics, Centers for Disease Control and Prevention, www.cdc.gov/nchs/products/vsus /vsus_1890_1938.htm.

153 *interview with the Holocaust survivor*: Elie Wiesel, "The Tragedy of the Believer," interview by Krista Tippet, *On Being*, July 13, 2006, https:// onbeing.org/programs/elie-wiesel-the-tragedy-of-the-believer.

165 *The late physician Paul Brand*: Philip Yancey and Paul Brand, *Fearfully and Wonderfully Made* (Grand Rapids: Zondervan, 1997), 68.

13 REFLECT

168 *a human matryoshka*: The concept, and some of the examples, are gleaned from Cristina Mazzoni, *Maternal Impressions: Pregnancy and Childbirth in Literature and Theory* (Ithaca, NY: Cornell University Press, 2002).

168 *In the Massachusetts Bay Colony*: Palmer Findlay, *Priests of Lucina: The Story of Obstetrics* (Boston: Little, Brown, 1939), 345.

171 *that patent lie that a woman's body can't*: Rep. Todd Akin (R-Missouri) effectively ended his campaign with his references to "legitimate rape" and his assertion that the "female body has ways to try to shut that whole thing down." The following article discusses some of the possible sources of this assertion: Tim Townsend, "Akin Appears to Have Picked Up Conclusions from 1972 Article Now Hotly Disputed," *St. Louis Post-Dispatch*, August 21, 2012, www.stltoday.com/news/local/metro/akin-appears-to-have -picked-up-conclusions-from-article-now/article_f267f02f-c9eb -515d-9a42-201de9b92d64.html.

172 *rates of abortion correlate highly with poverty*: See "Induced Abortion in the United States," Guttmacher Institute, www.guttmacher.org /fact-sheet/induced-abortion-united-states.

making it illegal does little: See Elisabeth Rosenthal, "Legal or Not, Abortion Rates Compare," *New York Times*, October 12, 2007, www.nytimes.com/2007/10/12/world/12abortion.html.

14 GROAN

182 *The diaries of the informally trained Maine midwife*: Laurel Thatcher Ulrich, *A Midwife's Tale: The Life of Martha Ballard Based on Her Diary (1785-1812)* (New York: Random House, 1990), 185, 188, 189.

187 *happy female socialization buzzing around births*: Sheila Kitzinger, *Rediscovering Birth* (London: Pinter & Martin, 2011).

Hmong culture prescribes a specific postpartum menu: Anne Fadiman, *The Spirit Catches You and You Fall Down* (New York: Farrar, Strauss & Giroux, 1997), 9.

189 *Food is treated as another unpleasant substance*: in Wendell Berry, *The Art of the Commonplace: The Agrarian Essays of Wendell Berry* (Berkeley, CA: Counterpoint, 2002), 151.

190 *good to* think: Claude Lévi-Strauss, quoted in Michael Pollan, *The Omnivore's Dilemma: A Natural History of Four Meals* (New York: Penguin Books, 2007), 289.